Sum of the Parts

Why Focusing on Diet and Weight Loss Alone Is a Losing Strategy for Better health

Jesse Lang PT

DEDICATION

This book is dedicated to all the hard-working individuals
who have tried diet after diet with limited success.

CONTENTS

ACKNOWLEDGMENTS

I would like to thank my mother. Her relentless focus on healthy foods and healthy living when I was growing up laid the foundation for my current lifestyle. This book would not have been possible without her.

INTRODUCTION

Bill and Carol recently retired. They had successfully run a wine and liquor store for 25 years in Nantucket and looked forward to spending their retirement enjoying their grandchildren, RV'-ing across the country, and cooking great meals at home. However, a major problem lay ahead of them that might alter their plans: their health wasn't where they wanted it to be.

At age 55, they both were fairly young for retirement, but they didn't feel young. Bill, whose long hours at the wine store had taken their toll on his body, had developed chronic back pain. Now, his back pain hurt him in the morning, it hurt him going up stairs, and most especially whenever he engaged in any lifting activities. Carol, on the other hand, didn't suffer from back pain as severely, but she had her own health issues, ranging from being overweight, to varicose veins, to mild psoriasis, and general arthritis. At a recent checkup, both Carol and Bill had been informed of slightly elevated cholesterol numbers, and had resisted the doctor's advice to start medication. They were now faced with the task of improving their health in order to ensure a healthy and long retirement, free from pain and disease. The only question remaining - was how to best accomplish this.

1 HAPPINESS AND WEIGHT LOSS

Carol and Bill were having dinner one evening at 8:30, when Carol mentioned to Bill that she had heard of a new podcast from her friend which seemed to be exactly what they were both looking for regarding their health questions. This podcast, called *Sum of the Parts*, was a comprehensive step-by-step guide to transforming your entire health for the long-term future. It didn't rely on fads or gimmicks, nor did it promote any trendy products such as oils, high-protein processed foods, or hypnosis. It was hosted by a licensed physical therapist who had 11 years of health-related university education, and several publications. He focused on research-based approaches that relied on recent discoveries in behavioral science, in order to transform bad habits into healthy habits that would lead to lasting health. He explained these concepts using simple analogies, allowing the listener to truly understand the *why* behind each new habit. While there is no perfect solution, Carol's friend highly recommended that

1

Carol and Bill give *Sum of the Parts* a shot, since it was free and was only 20 minutes once a week.

Bill wasn't a huge fan of podcasts, but when Carol mentioned they could listen to them in the RV during those times when the radio reception wasn't good, Bill agreed that it wouldn't be a huge sacrifice. He preferred the idea of listening to a podcast and working on a few habits as opposed to attending seminars or a loud gym with bright colors and complicated machines.

First Podcast

Follow me on a short journey. The journey is to happyland, a land where all humans want to live. Every person spends many years finding the correct directions to happyland, hoping that they will end up in the right place. Time and again though, when they arrive at the destination they typed into their smartphone or GPS device, they just see a bunch of other people in their cars, looking around confused. This journey never seems to reach the destination they seek.

The truth is that happyland is not a destination. There is no final place where one arrives and is continuously happy. I know of no one who achieved happiness by seeking happiness. Rather, happiness is a result of a life well lived, a life lived with purpose and meaning, with generosity, with loving and reciprocal relationships, with a satisfying and fulfilling career, and with health and peace of mind. Happiness will find those individuals who are living this way—it is truly that simple.

Now to weight loss. Weight loss, like happiness, is

not a destination. Those who seek to find weight loss by typing in various directions into their GPS devices will find themselves surrounded by other confused individuals, and without the desired results. I know of no one who achieved a lasting ideal weight by pursuing weight loss. Rather, weight loss is a result of a healthy life, filled with adequate and quality sleep, with good nutrition, regular physical activity, with low stress levels, and loving relationships. Ideal weight will find those individuals who are living this way; it is truly that simple.

Thank you for reading this book. I admire and respect you for caring enough to pursue a healthy life through evidence-based knowledge and for avoiding the fads and gimmicks that promise fast results with little sacrifice. I truly believe that if you follow the steps laid out in this book, you will become a healthier and happier person who will be living the life you have long envisioned for yourself. Please continue your journey and try to help others who are struggling to attain the same enlightenment that you will soon achieve.

Bill and Carol's Thoughts

The first podcast was short, and Bill liked that. It was right to the point. It made a very simple analogy that clearly showed what everyone knows, that seeking weight loss is the wrong strategy. While Bill hadn't focused on weight for most of his life like Carol had, ever since his back pain had started occurring, it seemed like all the doctors could focus on was his weight. Bill certainly had a gut, and trying to shrink it had seemed like a losing battle.

Furthermore, following Carol on every hair-brained diet scheme she had tried over the years had always seemed doomed to failure from the start. Bill didn't know if he was going to personally do anything different after this first podcast, but he enjoyed the ideas, and was happy to hear that it wasn't someone trying to sell him something.

For Carol, the first podcast had expressed what she had always known to be true, but perhaps due to the brainwashing that she'd received from every bit of media in her life, simply couldn't put into words. Of course, at the end of the day, Carol wanted to be healthy, not just thin. By focusing on weight loss, it was inevitable that other aspects of her health would be neglected, and now in her retirement years, the idea of sacrificing long-term health for short-term weight loss goals no longer appealed to her. She thought back to all of the diet fads she had lived through, and realized that they were all just schemes designed to take her money. Finally, here was someone telling her that focusing on weight loss was the wrong strategy, and that living a healthy life would bring her to her ideal weight naturally. What a refreshing concept this was!

2 WILLPOWER AND HABITS

Carol and Bill awoke in their RV in a campground in Arizona to a bright, sunny day. As Carol got dressed, she noticed her body in a new light. Today, she focused less on her belly and her soft spots, and a bit more on how she felt. She started to appreciate the lack of chronic back pain, and started to think about how she wanted her body to feel in the coming decades. Rather than focusing on beauty and thinness, she shifted her focus onto health and longevity. She was beginning to undergo a mental shift.

Bill wasn't experiencing the same mental shift, but he noticed that Carol wasn't criticizing her body the way she normally did. This was great for Bill, as Carol's weight had never really bothered him. Honestly, as far as Bill was concerned, as long as she paid attention to him and was intimate with him once a week, he was a happy camper. The more confident Carol was in her own body, the more attractive she became to Bill—five pounds here or there never mattered much to him.

Second Podcast

Willpower as a Muscle

Willpower—a word we often use, but we seldom stop to think about its meaning. What exactly is willpower? We know that some people seem to have lots of it while others have very little. We know that resisting urges and temptations requires a good amount of it, but have we ever thought about the role it plays in achieving the healthy lifestyle we all desire?

The best analogy is to think of willpower as a muscle. While not visible, the concept of willpower exists somewhere in our brains and it functions similarly to our muscles. Muscles, if used too much in a given day, begin to fatigue. When used excessively, they are unable to produce the same force as they were initially; no one can do an unlimited number of push-ups. Likewise, those who do push-ups regularly increase the size and strength of their muscles, enabling them to perform more push-ups than before. Doing one quick push-up or lifting something heavy once, however, will not build strength as effectively as doing multiple sets of a specific exercise. It is the details of how to effectively improve willpower that we are concerned with most.

Studies show that people who regularly practice religious acts have more willpower than those who do not.[1] Following on from this, people with greater willpower tend to be more financially successful than people who have little willpower.[2,3] Why? Because willpower is probably the single most important ingredient in determining whether you will be successful in achieving your goals. Willpower helps you to go to bed early, to avoid eating that candy bar, to work out consistently, and to clean the dishes before going to bed. Yet, we know that willpower is a limited resource and if we could find a way to increase the strength and stamina of our willpower then we would be more successful in achieving our goals.

How to Increase Willpower?

We have learned through research what works and what doesn't. What doesn't work are short bouts of intensely difficult decisions or situations that demand an immense amount of willpower: think torture. The victim is bound and forced to endure intense pain until he confesses his secrets. This activity requires a huge amount of willpower for a short period of time. A less dramatic activity still using up our willpower might be waiting in line at the post office for two hours. These activities, while depleting a great deal of willpower, do not strengthen it for the future. Instead, continual mindfulness, the kind that is required to maintain proper posture, is what really strengthens willpower. Other examples of activities that strengthen willpower include: routines, prayer, meditation, walking a dog daily, using your non-dominant hand for everyday tasks and several other activities. Think of these activities like doing a set of 20 push-ups. These activities use up some willpower, but they don't exhaust your willpower, and over time they become easier and easier to perform.

The Impact of Environment

While having strong inner willpower is critical to strictly maintaining one's behaviors, no person is immune to temptation. If, during a fast, you placed a bowl of chocolates on your desk while you worked, you would have to repeatedly use your willpower muscle to resist that temptation all day long. Eventually, that muscle would fatigue, and you would succumb to that temptation and break your fast. On the other hand, if a sex addict, looking to reform his ways, found himself on a deserted island, his problem would solve itself. These two examples illustrate how the power of our environment may either support or sabotage our willpower.

The beauty of our environment is that we can often control it. Looking to avoid fast food restaurants? Drive home from work through a different route that doesn't pass by McDonald's. Looking to work out more? Drive to and from work passing by your gym, or better yet, subscribe to a gym that is within eyesight of your home. Trying to quit smoking cigarettes? Remove all paraphernalia, clean your car and house from the smell of smoke, and stop frequenting bars and establishments where people who smoke are found.

Although not every aspect of our environment is able to be changed, modifying what we can in an effort to support our new behavior is a huge first step towards ensuring success in the future. This is just one reason why it is so important that both partners in a relationship be committed to a healthier lifestyle—because watching a partner fill up on sweets while viewing hours of TV from the couch will weaken your willpower over time.[4]

So the next time you go grocery shopping, think carefully about what you bring home. Even the strongest-willed people may weaken over time after seeing a chocolate eclair staring back at them every time they open the fridge.

The Problem with Setting Health Goals

We've all been told to set goals to achieve success, and even as children we are trained how to do this: get an A on this test, get into this college, get this degree, and then everything will work out for you. But why does this habit of setting goals lead us astray when we focus on our health?

Imagine a runner who sets a goal of running a marathon in four months. She will increasingly run longer and longer distances as she trains for the race, hopefully covering somewhere close to 23 miles in a single run a couple of weeks before the race. The focus and determination that is required when training for a marathon is immense, and naturally, most people are impressed when the runner crosses the finish line. But what happens after the marathon is over? Does the runner maintain her strict training regimen, or does she naturally relax back to her status quo?

This same relaxing back to the status quo occurs with health goals. When we first set a goal of losing 30 pounds in three months, for example, we become focused, just like the marathon runner. Looking towards that goal keeps us locked in, and allows us to stick to a difficult daily regimen. But as soon as we achieve that goal we naturally want a break, and we slowly return to our status quo. It is the act of setting a goal that will create this strict adherence, followed by the relaxing of our focus, which ultimately results in a less-than-healthy *you* in the future. Learning to live a healthier life every day, without the yo-yoing associated with setting health goals, is the surest way to achieve lifelong health.

Know the WHY to Endure Any HOW

Friedrich Nietzsche once said that if you know the *why*, you can endure any *how*. What does that really mean? It means that when you truly know the reason for why you want to accomplish or achieve something, then you will be able to endure whatever is necessary to achieve it. For example, if someone wants to quit smoking but isn't entirely sure of what their *why* is, then they will be less likely to endure the *how*, which in this case is the host of physical and mental hurdles inherent in nicotine addiction. If that person instead truly understands his *why*, that he wants to be alive to see his granddaughter graduate from high school, then he would be prepared to endure the ensuing *how*.

In the world of health and goal-setting, the rewards of our efforts are often far away and long awaited. We are not rewarded concretely on a daily basis for choosing the salad over the sandwich, but rather, these actions accumulate to produce a trimmer waistline, better complexion, and of course a lower risk of disease over time. In a world where everyone wants to be healthy, but few people are successful in following a healthy lifestyle without significant setbacks, we need to hone in on our *why*, and keep it close at hand. We need to think hard about our future, about our children, and perhaps about our grandchildren. Setting a goal of wanting to live to be 90 years old so that you can travel to Paris with your grandchildren is tangible. Putting a picture of your grandchildren and Paris on the fridge will help keep this *why* ever present in your mind, and remind you why you are enduring the *how*.

Actions you can take to improve your willpower today:

1. Create a morning routine that is fairly consistent and stick to it.
2. Go to bed and wake up roughly at the same time each day.
3. Make your own coffee, rather than purchase it from a store, and do this every day.
4. Take some time each morning to reflect on the day ahead, plan out what you want to achieve, and how you will achieve it.
5. If you are religious, put aside some time each day for prayer or religious thought or meditation and try to do this at the same time each day.
6. Focus on your posture and try to maintain proper posture throughout the day.
7. Prepare, cook, or bake some type of food on a regular basis.
8. If you do not already have one, create a financial budget and stick to it.
9. Introduce some type of daily physical activity, whether it be yard work, running, or something else that you enjoy.

10. Read a book or listen to an audiobook or podcast that you can learn something from for at least ten minutes each day.

How to Change Habits

Having strong willpower is certainly an advantage when seeking to change long-held habits. But strong willpower alone is insufficient—you must also have a strategy. The strategy for changing a habit is quite simple to understand, but more difficult to perform.

A habit has three major components: a cue or trigger, the routine or unwanted behavior, and the reward or outcome.[5] The way to successfully change a habit is to keep the cue and reward the same, while substituting a more desirable routine. We will break this down into simple steps using a sample habit of eating an entire pint of ice cream every night.

Step one: Identify your cues or triggers for the habit. Cues are usually location, time, hunger, an emotional state such as boredom or frustration, or a physical experience like cold, pain, or sex. Let's say your cue in the habit of eating a pint of ice cream is that *The Tonight Show* comes on. Every time it comes on, you get up, grab a pint of ice cream from the freezer, and continue to eat the entire pint while watching the show, until it is empty. It could just as easily be hunger, or boredom, or the time being 11:30, but in this case we will assume it is the television show. Once you identify the cue or trigger, you can move on to the reward.

Step two: Identify the reward for the habit. The reward could come in a variety of forms such as physical, emotional, or mental. For example, if you were hungry, the reward could be a cessation of the hunger, or feeling satisfied. The reward could also be the wonderful flavors of the ice cream, such as sugar and cream and chocolate. Or the reward could be the dopamine rush that accompanies the high-fat, high-sugar snack. If the reward is unclear at first, then you must move on to step three.

Step three: Start substituting different routines and see which ones continue to provide you with an adequate reward. For example, instead of eating a pint of ice cream, what if you just ate one quarter of the container? Do you still feel content and happy, or are you still craving that remaining three quarters? If you are still craving it, then try a different routine. What if you substituted a different food, such as a slice of watermelon, instead of the ice cream? Does this satisfy your craving and leave you feeling satisfied? If not, then continue to try other foods. But what if other foods don't provide you with the same sense of satisfaction? Perhaps the ice cream is providing you with such a strong dopamine rush, with its very high levels of sugar and fat, that no healthier food will suffice? In this case you may want to experiment with things other than food. Maybe calling a friend and laughing about something will help give you as much dopamine as the ice cream did. Perhaps playing with a pet outside would work. Maybe a brisk walk or even some intimate activity would be adequate. The point is to experiment with various alternate routines, until you are satisfied with the replacement routine. Once this is found, move onto the next step.

Step four: Reinforce the new habit. This may consist of you thinking about why you wanted to change this habit in the first place, such as losing excess weight, or saving the money you spent on ice cream weekly. Whatever the initial reason, now is the time to remind yourself of the *why* behind this behavior change. The other task is to highlight the rewards of the newly improved behavior. For example, put the money you would have spent on ice cream pints each week into a savings account and buy something for yourself. Or, save this money for a vacation at the end of the year. Whatever you do, be sure to enjoy the fruits of your new habit.

Step five: Have an emergency plan. Most new habits only last until the next major stressful event in one's life. During a major stressor, we revert to our old habits, as our willpower becomes depleted, and more of our actions become automatic. It is important to have a stress-relief emergency plan to turn to when something major occurs in our life. For example, if a loved one passes away, we need to turn to this plan and begin implementing the strategies that will decrease our stress and restore a calm peace to our life. As long as our stress levels remain elevated, the chance of reverting back to our old habits is high. Your emergency stress plan may consist of breathing and relaxation exercises, talking or meeting up with friends and family, exercising, or hitting a heavy bag. Whatever it is, have this plan in place prior to the stressful event occurring, so that when it does you are not *re*-acting, but *pro*-acting.

With a strong willpower muscle, a solid strategy to change your habit, and the willingness to do some hard work and experimentation, you should be able to change any unwanted habit you have to a healthier one.

Bill and Carol's Thoughts

This second podcast was a lot to digest. It was packed with information, and even better, it contained clearly outlined steps to take right now, without spending any money on bogus products or shakes. The hard part now was sticking to these new habits and staying consistent.

The step-by-step breakdown of how to specifically change a habit sounded vaguely familiar, but it was so clearly laid out this time that it seemed easier than ever. Both Carol and Bill had developed plenty of bad habits throughout their life, and now they had a clear strategy of how to replace these habits with better ones. Carol's habit that she would work on first would be her online shopping. First, she would find herself just looking at different items online, then adding them to her shopping bag, just to see the shipping cost, etc. Sooner or later, she'd find herself checking out and in a few days a package would arrive with her new item. Obviously, living according to a budget was essential, and she had purchased a few items she knew she really didn't need. But now, armed with a strategy to contain this habit, she felt confident that she could identify the trigger, and replace the shopping with a different action that would give her similar rewards.

Bill had many bad habits that he needed to work on, but he was going to start on his obsession with fantasy football. At first, it was just an occasional distraction during his week. He might spend 30 minutes picking his team and reviewing last week's results. But each year he had devoted more time and thought to this game, with no real earnings to show for it. He knew he could better spend this time on a number of other projects, and that four hours a week researching players and matchups seemed like a lot of time to be staring at a computer screen. So he would start applying the strategy to this habit, and slowly replace it with something more productive. He might not quit fantasy football altogether, but he'd restrict it to no more than 30 minutes a week.

Regarding willpower, Carol liked the part about the impact of environment. She knew all too well how difficult following her diets in the past had been, while watching Bill eat ice cream on the couch at night. Hearing the podcast tell her that exposing herself to these temptations actually depleted her willpower made all the sense in the world. Moving forward, Bill and Carol would be working together towards their health goals, and whatever foods or routines Carol was working on, Bill would be doing the same. This way, they would be a unified team, bolstering each other, rather than two distinct people who were often hindering each other's progress.

Bill found the part about health goals to be particularly enlightening. While he didn't know if he fully agreed yet, it had certainly made him think. He knew many of his friends who would tell him about a lofty health goal they had made, only to hear about how they'd slid right back as soon as the goal had been achieved. He remembered one friend in particular who had wanted to run a marathon before he turned 50. Yet, looking at him now, he was heavier than ever, and with an ankle injury from that race that still lingered to this day. The idea that most goals are mostly short-term motivating factors that lose their motivating ability once they are achieved made sense. But reorganizing one's mind around being healthy without using traditional goals still seemed abstract.

To Carol, the idea of goals as being unhelpful made more sense. She had achieved numerous weight loss goals throughout her life, only to slide inevitably back to her pre-diet weight, and sometimes even heavier. She explained to Bill that achieving a goal was a false victory. The willpower required to achieve the goal became depleted, and when you took a break from your training regime, your habits would revert back into easy and lazy ones. She suggested that what the podcast was probably trying to tell them was to pay more attention to their bodies on a minute-to-minute and daily basis, rather than using objective numbers to inform them of their status.

The part about knowing the *why* was very clear to both Bill and Carol: to spend as much time with their children and grandchildren as possible. They both wanted to see their grandchildren graduate from college and hopefully get married. Even though they only had two grandchildren, a boy named Edward, aged three, and a girl named Felicia, aged two, they were confident that this *why* was well worth enduring the *how*. They had pictures of their children and grandchildren displayed all throughout their RV and their home, and now when they looked at them, they were reminded of why they were working so diligently towards better health.

Immediately, Carol set to work implementing some new habits that would lead to greater willpower for both of them. She drove to the nearest supermarket and picked up some whole coffee beans, fresh produce, and a leg of lamb. Carol pulled out her coffee grinder and old French press that she hadn't used in years, and started making her own fresh coffee again. Within minutes, the aroma filled the RV, and she was floored at just how fragrant freshly ground coffee beans were. She then set to work chopping and dicing her produce in preparation for some braised lamb with roasted Brussels sprouts and bulgur. She had always enjoyed cooking, but had fallen into the routine of simple, quick meals that relied partially on processed, ready-made foods. She knew this had been the right way to eat from the beginning, and now that she realized this was actually improving her willpower, she applied herself with more energy than before.

Despite being only mildly religious, Carol had always enjoyed meeting new people at church, and also enjoyed going out to brunch with Bill afterwards. Therefore, they decided they would again resume the practice of attending church on Sundays, as a means to both bolster their willpower and be more social.

Regarding some of the other items on the willpower list, they already had a budget that Carol did monthly. Bill, on the other hand, had numerous back exercises that he was supposed to work on every day, but often forgot to do so for weeks at a time. Carol made a deal with Bill that she would clean the dishes if he would do his back exercises each night. Bill thought it was a good deal, and so they were in agreement. They were well on their way towards strengthening their willpower muscle for the challenges ahead.

References

1. McCullough, Michael E., and Brian LB Willoughby. "Religion, Self-regulation, and Self-Control: Associations, Explanations, and Implications." *Psychological Bulletin* 135.1 (2009): 69.
2. Metcalfe, Janet, and Walter Mischel. "A Hot/Cool-System Analysis of Delay of Gratification: Dynamics of Willpower." *Psychological Review* 106.1 (1999): 3.
3. Baumeister, Roy F., John Marion Tierney, and Denis P. O'Hare. *Willpower.* Simon & Schuster Audio, 2011.
4. Gorin, Amy, et al. "Involving Support Partners in Obesity Treatment." *Journal of Consulting and Clinical Psychology* 73.2 (2005): 341.
5. Duhigg, Charles. *The Power Of Habit: Why We Do What We Do In Life And Business.* New York: Random House, 2012. Print.

3 HOMEOSTASIS

After they had been working on the willpower activities for the past week, Bill and Carol were starting to feel more confident about their long-term health. Most of the changes they made to their activities had only been minor so far, and Bill had to admit that doing the exercises for his back regularly had allowed him to take less pain medication than normal. Carol and Bill both realized that their habits of online shopping and fantasy football were triggered by boredom, respectively, and found that replacing that activity with talking on the phone to friends and family gave them the same reward. Soon, they'd be saving money and building stronger relationships by swapping out better habits. They both agreed that their freshly made French-press coffee was better than the coffee from the Keurig, and it made the RV smell like a coffee shop in the morning. The church trip was a great opportunity for Carol to connect to the community and it also informed her indirectly of an antique sale nearby that she didn't know about previously. Bill preferred the brunch after church better, but it was a good feeling to be up and about on a Sunday morning rather than loafing around until noon either way. All in all, they hadn't had to give up anything they loved on this health journey yet.

Third Podcast

Knock Knock, It's Your Body

Knock knock. Who's there? It's your body. Your body who? Exactly. Unfortunately, most of us have forgotten how to listen to our bodies, or don't realize that our bodies are trying to communicate with us at all. But the truth is that our bodies are talking to us every day, all day long, and giving us most of the information that we need in order to make healthier decisions.

Imagine taking a school test but never receiving a grade. You wouldn't know if you were doing a good job. You wouldn't know whether you had actually learned the material or whether you were flunking the class. In the same sense, we need to know what effects our actions have on our body. We need to know if eating fast food makes us feel lethargic and mentally cloudy an hour later. If we ignore the information that our body sends to us, we won't know what effects our actions have on our health; this dialogue between us and our bodies needs to be opened.

But how do we listen to our bodies? Carefully, and mindfully. Listening to our bodies takes some effort, and a bit of willpower, but all of the information is there. We need to pay attention to the details of how we feel and be honest about how our actions may have created that feeling. How did drinking that extra glass of wine 20 minutes before bed affect you? Ask your body - Do you feel rested this morning? Do you feel cloudy? Chances are, your body will let you know that the glass of wine disrupted your sleep and that you feel a little cloudy the next day. How did that run affect your body? Later in the day you may have experienced a mental clarity and focus that you hadn't experienced in days. By paying attention to your body, you can determine if what you are doing is helping or hurting it.

The Limits of Repair

Our body is a living, breathing organism that can self-repair and restore itself. We can heal wounds, make scabs and scars, regrow skin, and perform a host of other amazing feats. We sometimes take for granted just how amazing our bodies are until they no longer work the way they're supposed to, and then we would trade anything to have those young restorative abilities back. But, aside from genetics, what allows some people to seemingly proceed throughout life without accumulating any real injuries and wounds, while others appear to be aging at double speed?

Briefly ignoring the countless factors that contribute to aging, let's focus on the balance between injury and repair. Imagine a well-maintained car that receives its services at every scheduled interval. It continues to run well, with the technicians repairing the small wear and tear that occurs from regular use. They change the oil, rotate the tires, and make sure all the fluids are clean. But what happens if you wait too long for a service? What if you forget to change your oil for 20,000 miles when the recommended interval is 7,500? The result may be permanent damage that cannot be undone by the technicians. Instead, you begin to see accelerated deterioration of your vehicle, and ultimately a shortened lifespan.

Similarly, our bodies can make small repairs each night. Have four or five beers, and your liver will process it eventually, and you may only have a mild headache for a couple of hours the next day. Smoke a couple of cigarettes once a week, and your lungs may be able to maintain their youthful elasticity for your full lifespan. Suntan for a couple of hours, and you may only have mildly inflamed skin for a day or two.

But overdo it, and your body cries "uncle." Once we push our bodies past this gentle elastic point, they can no longer repair us back to new, and we begin to age at an accelerated pace. After a night of binge drinking, there will be some mild brain damage and liver toxicity that cannot be undone.[1] Severely burn your skin after a day at the beach, and you will have just increased your chance of having skin cancer significantly.[2] These excesses can lead to one man looking 20 years older than he is, while his brother looks 20 years younger.

So next time you see someone who has great skin and looks ten years younger than their actual age, try to remember that our bodies have a limit to the amount of damage they can repair; overdo it, and you'll pay the price in the form of a shorter life.

Why Hydrating Is so Hard

Drink eight glasses of water. Drink two liters of water. Drink a half gallon of water. No matter how you slice it, we have all heard this mantra echoed again and again. Apparently, we don't drink enough water, and we're all walking around like dehydrated raisins, slowly killing our kidneys and impeding our metabolisms.

While I don't believe there is a set amount of water we should drink each day (it varies depending on a variety of factors), I do believe there are some reasons why we struggle to achieve adequate hydration.

Let's consider a car's oil. We all know that oil becomes dirty over time as flecks of debris and material accumulate. Also, some cars tend to burn oil, lowering the overall volume of oil and requiring periodic fill-ups. Either of these two processes will signal to the car's computer that there is a problem with the oil, causing the oil light to turn on.

Similarly, our thirst can generally be triggered by two processes: either an increase in the concentration of solutes (like salt and sugar) in our blood (this is analogous to dirty oil), or a reduction in the overall volume of our blood (analogous to burning oil).[3]

Under normal conditions where humans have access to water, this system is well regulated through our thirst signal, which stimulates us to drink water whenever one of the above two mechanisms occurs. But when certain additives are present, this can confuse the signals, making our thirst mechanism ineffective at regulating our hydration.

Looking back at the car analogy briefly, suppose

we add an "engine cleaner" additive that allegedly keeps the oil clean. While the truth of these claims is suspect, this additive can confuse the car's computer into thinking that the oil doesn't need to be changed as frequently as necessary. As a result, the car's oil may become dirtier than usual before the light comes on.

Similarly with humans, there are certain "additives" we can consume that will confuse our thirst signal, making it hard for us to stay hydrated properly. The most disruptive "additives" are alcohol, followed by high levels of caffeine.

When we consume alcohol we impair our kidneys' ability to conserve water. As a result, our blood becomes increasingly salty as we excrete dilute urine, and we begin to feel dehydrated. Similarly, caffeine in high levels (over 200ml) has a similar effect on our kidneys, again contributing to the feeling of dehydration.[3] Add in the consumption of salty foods and sugary drinks, which often accompany alcoholic beverages, and the resulting hangover from excessive dehydration is the obvious outcome.

Returning to the car analogy yet again, we see that older cars may be less effective at detecting when oil is dirty or needs to be topped up, as the sensors become defective or less sensitive. Similarly in humans, people over 50 years old have a decreased thirst signal, making their desire to drink water when they are dehydrated lower than in younger adults.[3]

To summarize, our hydration status may be compared to an engine's oil. Humans may detect dehydration through either an increase in salt and sugar in the blood, or a loss of plasma (excess sweating or blood loss). The signal to drink works fine for most younger adults, but not for older adults. Also, additives such as alcohol, caffeine, sugary drinks and salty foods can disrupt this system, leading to periods of dehydration that disrupt our day. Symptoms of dehydration include: lethargy (fatigue), weakness, irritability, increased muscle tension and edema (swelling).

The takeaway is that due to age and substances like alcohol and caffeine, we can no longer rely on our internal cues to properly regulate our hydration status.

Below is a list of ways that we can stay properly hydrated and avoid the unwanted symptoms of dehydration:

1. At a minimum, try to drink at least two liters of water per day for women and 2.5 liters of water per day for men.
2. Water is not appealing to everyone, so choose something that you enjoy drinking. Seltzer with natural flavors and scents works well. Also, adding lemon or lime juice to water can improve the palatability for some people. Diluted fruit juices (85% water, 15% juice) can provide just enough sugar to stimulate adequate consumption for hydration.
3. Avoid highly concentrated beverages such as undiluted fruit juice, energy drinks, or soda as a replacement for water. Even sugar-free beverages contain artificial sweeteners which can decrease their hydrating effect.[4]
4. Limit the amount of caffeine you consume to a reasonable amount. The exact amount may vary depending on your previous intake, body weight and metabolism, but over 400ml of caffeine will contribute to dehydration.[5]

5. Limit the amount of alcohol you consume. Obviously, people will continue to consume large quantities of alcohol, but try to stop drinking two hours before bedtime and have at least 20 oz. of water before you go to bed. This will help to mitigate some of the dehydration you will experience the next day.

6. Limit the amount of salty foods you consume. Today's packaged foods nearly all contain higher amounts of salt than foods found in nature or prepared at home. If you love your salt, just keep in mind that you will need to drink an even greater amount of water to compensate.

7. Use your urine as an indicator of hydration status. Your urine should be pale yellow to clear. Dark orange or brown urine is an indicator of dehydration.[6]

8. Listen to your body to assess hydration status. Does your skin feel tight? Does your mouth feel dry? Are your eyes drier than usual? As you become attuned to these parts of your body you may be able to sense when you are running low on fluids.

9. Drink more than you think you need to when exercising in the cold. Cold weather dampens your sense of thirst, despite you needing water.[7] Next time you shovel the driveway or go skiing, think about rehydrating *before* you feel thirsty.

Bill and Carol's Thoughts

This most recent podcast had a bit more science to it, which wasn't Carol and Bill's specialty. Nevertheless, the car analogy made a lot of sense to Bill, so he was able to understand the science completely by the end of the podcast. Hydration status was not something he had really thought about on a daily basis, so this podcast certainly made him start thinking about water in a different light. He had to admit that he wasn't drinking 2.5 liters of water each day, and liked the idea of drinking seltzer with a splash of cranberry and a lime as a way to increase his consumption of fluids. Carol had been more aware of her water intake, as many of her previous diets had extolled the virtues of staving off hunger by drinking more water. But even Carol admitted that she would forget about her water intake during the colder months, and forgot to adjust for alcohol and caffeine intake.

The information about avoiding alcohol before bedtime and excess caffeine and salt made the most sense. Carol and Bill had begun avoiding Chinese food recently, as they both would wake up feeling hungover as a result of the excessive salt used in the food. Enjoying this food earlier in the evening, and then following it with several ounces of water might be the solution to their Chinese-food-hangover episodes. Also, Bill enjoyed a couple of beers each night and sometimes a glass of Scotch or bourbon before bed. He said it helped him to fall asleep, but admitted that he did seem a bit foggier the day after having this liquor right before bed. Shifting this alcohol intake to earlier in the evening and consuming some extra water before bed might allow Bill to continue to enjoy his spirits while avoiding this mental fog.

Carol particularly enjoyed the piece about listening to your body. This part of the podcast resonated with her. After following so many diets, she was tired of having someone else tell her what to eat and how to act. She felt that her body was wise enough to inform her of what foods and activities it needed and preferred. She wanted to be more independent with her dietary and exercise choices, and knew that the answer did not lie in the next weight-loss book or program, but rather within her own body's wisdom. She could detect when a certain food made her feel lethargic or bloated and would pay closer attention to these signals in the future. Further, she also knew that certain foods gave Bill heartburn, and seemed to negatively affect his sleep. Knowing that the answer to many of her questions lies within her own body, Carol felt more confident and independent in her journey towards a healthier life.

The next steps they needed to take to start applying this week's lessons were clearly spelled out for them. First, they would both have water bottles with them wherever they went. Nothing fancy, just durable bottles that were easily opened, easily cleaned, and held at least 20 ounces of fluid. Next, they would stock up on seltzer, cranberry juice cocktail, and a few limes. Armed with their mildly flavored beverages, Bill and Carol were confident that their fluid consumption would increase. Since they now brewed their own coffee, they decided to opt for darker roasts, since these contained less caffeine than lighter roasts. Higher caffeine levels could contribute to dehydration. Paying attention to urine color and skin turgor was an easy and quick way to determine hydration status. Carol knew that she drank less fluids during the colder months, so she would try to keep this information in mind when winter approached. Armed with these few small changes, and a mindset of paying closer attention to their bodies, Carol and Bill felt well prepared to embrace the challenge of maintaining their bodies in a healthy homeostasis.

References

1. Ward, Roberta J., Frédéric Lallemand, and Philippe De Witte. "Biochemical and Neurotransmitter Changes Implicated in Alcohol-Induced Brain Damage in Chronic or 'Binge Drinking' Alcohol Abuse." *Alcohol and Alcoholism* 44.2 (2009): 128-135.
2. MacKie, Rona M. "Long-Term Health Risk to the Skin of Ultraviolet Radiation." *Progress in Biophysics and Molecular Biology* 92.1 (2006): 92-96.
3. Turner, Neil, et al. *Oxford Textbook of Clinical Nephrology.* Oxford University Press, 2015.
4. Martínez, Claudia, et al. "Effects on Body Mass of Laboratory Rats after Ingestion of Drinking Water with Sucrose, Fructose, Aspartame, and Sucralose Additives." *Open Obes J* 2 (2010): 116-24.
5. Robertson, David, et al. "Effects of Caffeine on Plasma Renin Activity, Catecholamines and Blood Pressure." *New England Journal of Medicine* 298.4 (1978): 181-186.
6. Mentes, Janet C., Bonnie Wakefield, and Kennith Culp. "Use of a Urine Color Chart to Monitor Hydration Status in Nursing Home Residents." *Biological Research for Nursing* 7.3 (2006): 197-203.
7. Kenefick, ROBERT W., et al. "Thirst Sensations and AVP Responses at Rest and During Exercise-Cold Exposure." *Medicine and Science in Sports and Exercise* 36.9 (2004): 1528-1534.

4 STRESS

Bill and Carol awoke to a crisp spring morning. Today was a good day, and it was also the day of the next podcast installment. Carol was enjoying this journey towards a healthier life. She had already started noticing improvements in the way she felt. For example, she used to wake up from sleeping with a dry mouth, and occasionally a faint headache. But after the tweak to her fluid intake, she would wake up feeling hydrated and found it easier to begin her day. She used to need coffee immediately for a jump-start, but now that she was fully hydrated, she felt less reliant on caffeine.

Bill also, found that by shifting his alcohol intake to earlier in the evening, the mental fogginess the next day had almost disappeared. While he was still getting used to carrying a water bottle around with him at all times, he didn't mind the seltzer/cranberry-lime mixture, and had discovered that the activity of drinking water reminded him of his other healthful habits. It was as if by paying attention to his hydration levels, he was also paying more attention to his body and how he was feeling. For example, Bill noticed that now that he was fully hydrated, his back pain was more manageable than before. As his hydration status improved, the volume of his vertebral discs increased, providing more room for his vertebrae and nerves to move past each other; small steps were leading to big changes.

Fourth Podcast

What Is Stress?

Stress may refer to a number of things, but in terms of health we are talking mainly about the state that the body is in when it is unable to maintain homeostasis. In other words, stress is what happens when something from the external environment disrupts our physiological balance to the point that it produces negative physical or mental effects. The opposite of stress would be a coma, where the body is sort of in a completely stable state, being unaffected and unchanged by the environment.

With stress defined, let's examine what type of stress is harmful to us. Two factors should be considered: duration and intensity. Very intense stressful moments may only last a few seconds (a police car in your rearview mirror), and these are not very harmful. Likewise, very low intensity stress may last for days (breaking in a new pair of shoes), and these moments are also not very harmful. We are most concerned with stress that is of somewhat modest intensity but also that lasts for weeks and months (being the president of a country, for example), and what the effects of this may be on our health. Mathematically, multiplying the intensity by the duration gives us the total "stress load" on the body.

The short-term effects of stress are well understood and written about extensively elsewhere. I will briefly describe them here. Think of the Mouse Trap game, which uses a series of linked actions, to visualize what happens in our body. The hypothalamus, located in our midbrain, senses a change to the state of the body, be it temperature, pain, thirst, etc. This triggers a series of chemical reactions, which lead to the release of norepinephrine and cortisol, in the brain and body, respectively. The short-term effects of these chemicals are elevated heart rate, elevated blood pressure, dilated pupils, redistribution of blood from digestive organs to muscles, and the numerous other physical effects we've come to associate with the fight-or-flight response.[1] These two chemicals that cause the short-term effects of stress are also largely responsible for the long-term effects of chronic stress as well.

One negative effect of chronic stress is on immune function. Cortisol is a master switch for our immune system, and when it remains elevated for a long period of time it suppresses our immune cells' ability to multiply and divide. It also hinders the chemical messengers, called cytokines, which help the immune system to ramp up its defenses in response to a foreign invader. This is why we are more likely to become sick during periods of prolonged stress. Furthermore, cortisol has additional negative effects on our bodies, such as impaired wound healing, decreased growth hormone production, decreased responsiveness of our hypothalamus, and increased visceral fat deposition, to name a few.[2]

Between cortisol and norepinephrine, some of the combined effects of chronic stress include: increased blood pressure, increased risk of cardiovascular accidents, increased anxiety and depression, decreased fertility, and an overall acceleration of the aging process.[2] If only there was some way we could intervene to reset our hypothalamus and minimize the effects of stress on our health...

Stress-O-Stat

Think of your stress level like the thermostat in your house, a stress-o-stat, if you will. Just like a thermostat, a stress-o-stat dictates the level of stress you experience on a daily basis. When the temperature in your house becomes too warm, you turn down the thermostat and the temperature drops. We know how to adjust our thermostat, but what if we could adjust our stress level in the same way? Well, we can—and anyone can do it. The best part is that it's completely free and something that we all know how to do: slow breathing.

What does slow breathing mean? Simply put, breathing between two to four times each minute for 20 minutes per day. Slow inhale, hold briefly, slow exhale, hold briefly, repeat. The slower you breathe, the greater the reduction in stress will be. The results, while not 100% immediate, will be lowered anxiety and stress, decreased heart rate, decreased blood pressure, improved digestion, improved sexual performance, and many more.[3,4,5] Mentally, you will once again be aware of your surroundings and have greater control over your thoughts. Controlling your thoughts directly is nearly impossible, but by breathing slowly, we are controlling our autonomic nervous system, and this will ultimately change the way our brain works. It is one of the few areas where an action will have a direct and positive effect on our thoughts.

When should you breathe slowly? Whenever it is most convenient for you, but at a time that you can remember to perform daily. I do my breathing during my commute to work. This is especially useful, since driving can sometimes trigger sympathetic activity, and breathing slowly tends to reduce the stress of that task. If you don't commute, then find some other time, perhaps during commercials between TV shows, using the bathroom, or while walking your pet. Whatever it is, just try to be consistent and accumulate at least 20 minutes of slow breathing each day. If you miss a day, don't worry, just resume as soon as you can. The great news: more slowed breathing can't hurt you, it will only lead to a calmer, less stressful you.

Armed with this new tool, you now have the ability to control your own stress-o-stat without the need for drugs or hypnotherapy. Begin today, and start to feel the stress literally melt away. You will be amazed at how much more energy you have when you aren't perpetually anxious.

Steps to slow breathing and reduced anxiety:

1. Slow breathing can be performed anytime, anywhere, for any period of time.

2. The goal is to achieve a total of 20 minutes of slow breathing each day.
3. Begin by inhaling slowly, for roughly four seconds.
4. Once fully inhaled, try to hold this for another four to six seconds.
5. Then, slowly exhale over eight to twelve seconds.
6. Repeat the process, trying to slow your breathing down to about four breaths per minute.
7. As you gain comfort with this, you can aim for even fewer breaths per minute, down to a goal of two breaths per minute if this is comfortable for you.
8. That's it! Now practice your slow breathing as much as possible in as many situations as you can and enjoy the rewards of decreased anxiety.

So, if That Is What Slow Breathing Does....Why Do We Yawn?

Nearly every person has wondered about the meaning of yawns. Why are they contagious? Why do I yawn at night when I'm tired but also before a test when I'm nervous? Why do animals yawn? I will reveal to you the common thread behind yawning, and how it gives us insight into our body's remarkable physiology.

Yawning, quite simply, is a way of slowing down our breathing. Think about it: a yawn causes you to stop your breathing, take a deep breath, keep your mouth agape for a few seconds, and then, when that wave of relief washes over you, it prompts a slow exhale. So, if we know that yawning slows down our breathing, what effect does this have on our bodies?

We already know that breathing is the knob on our body's stress-o-stat which controls the stress levels (sympathetic nervous system) of our body. By slowing our breathing, we decrease our sympathetic output and decrease our stress. The physical result is slowed heart rate, lower blood pressure and decreased anxiety, among other things.

Now back to yawning. We yawn to decrease our anxiety and put us in a state of relaxation. This is why we yawn when we are tired—it is our body's way of telling us to calm down and go to sleep. But what about the social contagiousness of yawning? This serves the function of signaling to other people that we feel safe around them and aren't threatened. If we yawn, we signal to the person that we are calm and not anxious, and this promotes social bonding; a slowed heart rate and decreased anxiety is beneficial for forming social bonds. Additionally, people like to have others mirror their body language. By yawning after another person has yawned, we strengthen the social bond between individuals.

So there you have it, yawning decreases our anxiety, calms us down to prepare us for sleep or reduce our anxiety, and has evolved to provide a social lubricating function by showing others that we are not threatened by them. Pretty cool, huh?

The Flipside of the Coin: Fast Breathing

It should follow logically that if slow breathing decreases anxiety, then fast breathing should increase anxiety. The good news is that this is true. Should fast breathing never be practiced then, and always be viewed as an unhealthy action? Not necessarily. For along with anxiety, fast breathing also ramps up the fight-or-flight systems in our body, many of which may be useful for various tasks and moments in our lives.

For example, when waking up in the morning, we often feel groggy and reach to hit the snooze button. If we instead perform ten deep, fast breaths, we may find that our blood flow has increased, our energy levels have risen, and we feel more alert and prepared to take on the new day. Likewise, if we are to perform a feat which requires some physical exertion and energy, a few deep and quick breaths may inject ourselves with the energy and focus that we need for such a task.

Instead of viewing slow breathing as the only useful type of breathing, learn to think of your breath as a tool that you can use to react to any given situation more easily. While the majority of us tend to experience too much anxiety, and long-term stress leads to numerous unwanted health outcomes, some people may lack sufficient energy and vigor for stressful events. These people may be better served by employing fast breathing as needed. The bottom line is that we can adjust our body's autonomic nervous system through breathing, putting the control back in our hands.

Anxiety and Sex

No book on health would be complete without mentioning sex, which is an important part of many people's healthy lives. After all, without sex, neither you nor I would be here today. But why discuss sex with anxiety? Why not in the chapter on happiness? Allow me to explain.

Recalling the first section of this chapter, our

homeostasis is largely determined by our hypothalamus. This region of the brain helps balance our autonomic nervous system and determines whether we are in "fight-or-flight" mode (sympathetic output) or "rest-and-digest" mode (parasympathetic output). These two phases of our nervous system affect multiple organs throughout the body, including the sex organs. The confusing part, is that men and women are affected differently by these systems.

Men: Anxiety is a death sentence for men as it relates to sex. If our sympathetic nervous system gets activated, all sorts of negative consequences can occur. To begin with, men must become aroused. This requires that they are fairly relaxed and calm initially. When the parasympathetic nervous system (PNS) is activated, blood flow is increased to the sexual organs, increasing the chance that an erection will occur. In order to maintain this erection, the man must avoid becoming too excited, or in other words, minimize the sympathetic nervous system's (SNS) contributions. If the SNS becomes activated, this will trigger an ejaculation, followed quickly by the loss of the erection, as the blood flow to the sexual organs diminishes. On the other hand, if the male is not stimulated enough, he may be unable to achieve an orgasm, and this is also an unwanted outcome.[6] Therefore, the careful balance between PNS and SNS output is essential to a successful sexual event.

Women: Anxiety plays a different role with women. Whereas anxiety will prevent a man from achieving and maintaining an erection, anxiety can actually increase sexual desire in women. PNS activity still increases blood flow to the genitalia, similarly to men, which may explain why a calm, sensual environment with lots of foreplay helps to get a woman started. But, since women don't need to maintain an erection like a man does, the more important function for most women is to be able to achieve orgasm. In this case, anxiety actually promotes orgasm for both the man and the woman.[7] Often, with men, a postponement of orgasm is desired, while with women, a hastening of the orgasm is desired. Thus, the sexes generally want two different mood states during sex: men seek less anxiety to prolong sex, and women seek more anxiety to promote orgasm. It is not a coincidence that books like *50 Shades of Grey* are so popular, as some women enjoy the fear/anxiety associated with dominating and sometimes slightly painful activities. A number of women enjoy some type of "rough play" such as choking, spanking or bondage, and since we now know that this anxiety can help some women achieve orgasm, it should come as no surprise.

The bottom line: Men should focus on slow breathing activities and try to keep anxiety to a minimum in order to promote longer and more sustainable sex; hence tantric sex focuses on slow-breathing exercises to prolong sexual activity. Meanwhile, women should try injecting some "rough play" or excitement into the bedroom in order to create some anxiety/fear that will help to promote an orgasm. Of course, everyone is different and there is no one rule for everyone, but this is generally how our bodies respond to anxiety as it relates to sex.

A Word on Digestion

"To eat is human, to digest, divine." This quote by Mark Twain highlights the simple principle that we now overlook, that proper digestion is a wonderful experience that often eludes the busy person. Snacks, drive-throughs, grab-and-goes, eating on the run, and any other form of rushed dining experience assumes that our digestive organs will be able to work their magic despite whatever else we are doing. We need to stop and consider what our body wants after we eat and pay more attention to extracting the full nutrients from our food, rather than viewing food as merely fuel.

Look at a lion after he eats. He isn't running around; rather, he's lying around, napping, scratching his face, and otherwise relaxing. Do you think it's a coincidence that we become sleepy after eating a large meal? We are supposed to relax after we eat so that our body can digest properly. The PNS (rest and digest) kicks into gear after a meal, increasing blood flow to our digestive organs and helping us to fully extract all the nutrients in our meal. If instead of relaxing we go right back to work, increasing our anxiety and our SNS activity (fight or flight), then blood flow will be directed *away* from our digestive organs. This stress or SNS activity also slows down the peristaltic motions of our organs and can lead to an increase of symptoms such as heartburn, indigestion, cramping, bloating, and constipation. It's no wonder that so many people now have irritable bowel syndrome (IBS), partly due to our hectic lifestyles.[8]

Furthermore, when we are not relaxed after eating,

we do not receive the same amount of nutrients from our food that we do when we are calm. Thus, a large meal full of fat and protein not only nourishes us less when we are stressed, but this lack of nourishment also makes our brain think that we need to eat more, since our body didn't receive all of the nutrients that it otherwise would have if we were relaxing.[9]

Lastly, eating should be one of life's great pleasures. By relaxing after we eat, we can truly enjoy the calm experience the way we were supposed to, and the more we enjoy our food, the less likely the dangerous habit of binge-eating is to occur.[10] If you aren't able to relax after eating at work, perhaps eating smaller meals during work would help, moving the larger meals to pre- or post-work when you have time to relax afterwards. Remember, anxiety and digestion are at odds with each other, so try to promote a calmer state after you eat. Your lack of heartburn and indigestion will be just one of the many rewards.

Mindfulness

Mindfulness is a word that is bandied around frequently these days. From yoga, to meditation, to cognitive behavioral therapy, it appears that mindfulness is the solution to everyone's problems. But before leaving this chapter on stress, let's discuss what mindfulness actually means and why it may be just as important as it seems.

First imagine a cat, lazily lying around. It seems like it has no worries in the world. It may feel thirsty or hungry from time to time, and so it lumbers over to the food bowl to satisfy these desires. Then the cat may want some warmth, so it lies on the floor in the sunlight. Later, it might be inclined to sit upon its owner's lap for some affection. What this cat doesn't realize, however, is that it is the embodiment of mindfulness. For it is in the absence of worries and faraway thoughts that we become mindful of the world and present situation around us.

Mindfulness is simply being present, immersing yourself in the moment, focusing on what you are doing at hand, and not thinking about other problems or situations that aren't here and now.

Research has shown that we are happiest when we focus on what we are doing. Even during a commute, an experience almost universally despised, thinking about being somewhere else makes us less happy than just focusing on elements in the car or the trees and landscape surrounding us. By thinking about being somewhere else, it causes a slight stress in our psyche that slowly erodes our happiness and accumulates in our body.[11] The antidote is to slow down, be present, and be mindful.

Bill and Carol's Thoughts

This podcast was a game-changer. Managing stress and anxiety had been such a struggle for Carol, especially when she was a working mother. She would worry and panic, and let her anxiety affect her sleep and her enjoyment of everyday events. Bill too, would often become stressed with his work, taking it too seriously, as well as succumbing to occasional fits of road rage when traversing the country in his RV. Now that they were retired it seemed slightly easier to manage their stress, but as their doctors had told them, managing their stress levels would have widespread health benefits.

Bill particularly enjoyed the idea of slow breathing compared to meditation. He had tried meditation numerous times in his life, with little success. Sitting in an uncomfortable position, sometimes surrounded by strangers, trying to think of nothing, was too abstract and unfamiliar. Slow breathing, on the other hand, was simple and straightforward. Bill spent long hours driving the RV, and knew that he would choose that time to focus on the slow breathing exercises.

Carol found the bit about yawning fun and interesting. It helped to reinforce the power of slow breathing, but she thought she might use it as a psychology barometer at social events to determine which people were very relaxed and which were anxious.

The bit about sex was fun, although not as relevant at this point in their relationship. Bill remembered when he was younger and anxious with a woman, how it would hinder his performance. He also remembers learning how some women enjoyed the "rough stuff" to some degree, and now it made sense to him from a physiologic standpoint. Carol felt that she didn't agree 100% with what stimulated women, but thought the information about men reinforced her underlying beliefs that they need to be relaxed and calm for sustained performance.

Indigestion had long been a concern for Bill. Like most Americans, he enjoyed his sausages, fried foods, and other fatty meats. But as he advanced in age, and slowly gained weight, he experienced more heartburn, especially when eating close to bedtime. He thought that part of the problem lay in going to these fast casual restaurants like Chili's and Applebees where you eat loads of greasy food quickly, followed by a dessert, and then rush out of the restaurant to make room for the next table. Now that Carol and he were preparing more food at home, they were able to slow down, have time between courses, and shift dessert to lunchtime, rather than trying to stuff it in after dinner. Bill loved to relax after a good meal, and he certainly noticed a difference in his indigestion when he was relaxed as opposed to running around.

The last bit about mindfulness again resonated with Carol soundly. She had really embraced listening to her body over the past week, and being told to be more present and mindful in the moment just helped to reinforce her new habits. Some of the best memories Carol had were when she had been on her sister's farm, pulling carrots from the field, washing them by hand, and carefully preparing the night's meal with care. These slow country nights seemed to epitomize "living well", and were moments when Carol truly felt connected to her body and her family. By slowing down and focusing on the moments, and enjoying food and company, she knew she could overcome many of the binges and other food relapses she had succumbed to in the past.

References

1. Robertson, David; Biaggioni, Italo; Burnstock, Geoffrey; Low, Phillip A; Paton, Julian F.R. *Primer On The Autonomic Nervous System 3rd Edition*. London: Academic Press, 2012. Print.

2. Melmed, Shlomo; Polonsky, Kenneth S; Larsen, P Reed; Kronenberg, Henry M. *Williams Textbook of Endocrinology 13th Edition*. Philadelphia: Elsevier, 2016. Print

3. Bernardi, Luciano, et al. "Slow Breathing Reduces Chemoreflex Response to Hypoxia and Hypercapnia, and Increases Baroreflex Sensitivity." *Journal of Hypertension* 19.12 (2001): 2221-2229.

4. Tang, Yi-Yuan, et al. "Central and Autonomic Nervous System Interaction is Altered by Short-Term Meditation." *Proceedings of the National Academy of Sciences* 106.22 (2009): 8865-8870.

5. Joseph, Chacko N., et al. "Slow Breathing Improves Arterial Baroreflex Sensitivity and Decreases Blood Pressure in Essential Hypertension." *Hypertension* 46.4 (2005): 714-718.

6. Andersson, Karl-Erik, and Gorm Wagner. "Physiology of Penile Erection." *Physiological Reviews* 75.1 (1995): 191-237.

7. Fisher, Seymour. *Understanding the Female Orgasm*. Basic Books, 1973.

8. Barrett, Kim E. *Gastrointestinal Physiology 2nd Edition*. New York: McGraw-Hill Education, 2014. Print.

9. David, Marc. *The Slow Down Diet: Eating for Pleasure, Energy & Weight Loss*. Rochester: Healing Arts Press, 2005. Print.

10. Kristeller, Jean, Ruth Q. Wolever, and Virgil Sheets. "Mindfulness-Based Eating Awareness Training (MB-EAT) for Binge Eating: A Randomized Clinical Trial." *Mindfulness* 5.3 (2014): 282-297.
11. Campos, Daniel, et al. "Meditation and Happiness: Mindfulness and Self-Compassion May Mediate the Meditation–Happiness Relationship." *Personality and Individual Differences* 93 (2016): 80-85.

5 SLEEP AND ENERGY LEVELS

Bill's doctor was surprised. Bill's heart rate had decreased from 85 beats per minute at his last check-up to 70 beats per minute on his most recent one. Additionally, his systolic blood pressure was nearly 10 mmHg lower as well. His doctor was so happy with this improvement that he decided to hold off on adding an anti-cholesterol drug, since whatever he was doing seemed to be showing some major improvements.

Of course, Bill knew what had caused the change, but didn't want to bore the doctor with all of the small changes he had made over the past four weeks. He was just happy that his actions were making a difference, and that he was well on his way towards a healthier and happier future. Recently, however, Bill had noticed how the slow breathing had calmed him down during his long drives, and he could even sense his heart rate slowing down throughout the week.

Carol too, had noticed some weight loss over the past four weeks. She had only lost two pounds, but the weird part is that she hadn't really been trying to lose weight. She was just following the podcasts and making small changes. She thought that the shift to eating dessert earlier, and making more of her meals at home were probably the biggest factors in her weight loss. But more important was that she felt she had more energy and less anxiety than in recent memory. For Carol, she was maturing past the goal of trying to "look fabulous" and instead wanted to feel healthy. So far, it had been working well.

Fifth Podcast

Why Do We Sleep?

Sleep is something we do every night—sometimes every other night—whether we want to or not, yet most of us know very little about it. For example, scientists don't definitively know *why* humans sleep, or any organism for that matter. But, certainty aside, let's examine the two main purposes for sleep with regards to our health, and what simple actions we can take to maximize the quality of the sleep we achieve each night.

So what is the reason we need to sleep? There are generally two reasons why sleep is important for us as humans. The first is to restore our physical body. This process roughly consists of rebuilding cells, repairing damage, building muscle and bone, refreshing our immune system, balancing our hormone levels and the routine maintenance of our body.[1] Think of sleep like a tune-up for our car. It makes sure that all the physical and mechanical systems of our body are running smoothly and efficiently, and ensures that we can drive on the road for quite some time before the wheels fall off, so to speak. Or another analogy could be the recharging of your smartphone; without a fully charged battery your phone will crash at some point during the day, just like your body falling asleep in the afternoon.

The second reason we sleep is to organize our brain. Think of our brain as a desk. Throughout a busy day our desk becomes cluttered with papers. Some of these papers are important, others are not. If we don't file these papers at the end of the day, then when we arrive at work the next day, we'll have a mess on our hands. If we continue to work without organizing our desk we will become inefficient and have trouble finding any file of importance, since it'll be buried in a pile of papers. Similarly, our brain accumulates information or files throughout the day that need to be organized. If we stored every piece of information we ever acquired, we would be unable to retrieve important information efficiently. By throwing out or deleting unnecessary information and condensing or organizing useful information, our brain is better positioned to learn new tasks and items and retrieve useful information quickly.

Another useful analogy is a computer that needs to be restarted once a week to continue to perform efficiently. If you use your computer for a week without restarting it, it begins to slow down, taking multiple seconds to perform tasks that previously only took fractions of a second. Thus, in order to keep our memory sharp and our learning capacity full, we need to sleep in order to allow this neural reorganization to occur.[2]

Effects of Insufficient Sleep

Now that we know *why* we need to sleep, let's briefly review what happens to both our bodies and our brains if we don't get enough sleep.

Physically: impaired immune function, increased heart rate variability, decreased reaction time, tremors, aches, decreased coordination, suppression of growth activities, increased risk of obesity, increased risk of type 2 diabetes and high blood pressure.[3]

Mentally: increased anxiety, increased irritability and general grouchy mood, impaired memory, shortened attention span and hallucinations, to name a few.[4]

How Much Should We Sleep?

Okay, so we now know the reason why we must sleep, and what happens if we don't get quality sleep. The next step is to determine how many hours we should be sleeping, and what we can do to make sure that those are quality hours.

The ideal amount of time for adults to sleep is generally between seven to nine hours.[5] With that being said, each person's ideal time may vary slightly, and the simple way to determine that will be described below.

Good Quality Sleep

With the ideal time addressed, what about quality sleep? What factors can impair quality sleep? Chemically, any type of stimulant that is still active when you go to sleep will interfere with the quality of sleep. These may include caffeine (active for up to 12 hours after consumption), nicotine, Ritalin (ADHD medication), methamphetamines, ephedrine, etc.[6] In addition to stimulants, numerous other chemical compounds such as alcohol, THC (cannabis), and many over-the-counter drugs can disrupt normal sleep patterns. What is more surprising is that even the types of food eaten close to bedtime can impair sleep quality.[7]

Regarding quality of sleep, it is interesting to note that in the first half of the night the body is largely addressing the physical aspects of sleep, whereas in the latter half of the night the body is addressing the mental or brain aspects of sleep. While both aspects are being addressed the entire time, there is a general shift from physical, restorative sleep during the first four hours, to mental organization and memory improvements during the latter half of sleep.[8]

What about naps? Good? Bad? Well, naps can be helpful if you need one, but there are specific guidelines to maximize their benefits, which are outlined below.

Lastly, how do we minimize that grogginess when we first wake up? This grogginess is called sleep inertia, and it can take two to four hours for it to clear, and for you to achieve your full mental clarity. Use of stimulants such as caffeine have been shown to decrease this grogginess while having minimal impact on sleep quality if taken with enough time between ingestion and bedtime.[9,10]

The Final Minutes

The final minutes before bedtime are perhaps the

most important minutes of your entire next day. This is the time when you will prepare yourself for either a relaxing sleep, or a night filled with interruptions and restlessness.

The first order of business is checking in on hydration levels. If you are dehydrated, make sure to drink water. There are few experiences worse than waking up in the middle of the night with a mouth that feels like the desert. In addition, even if you do sleep through the night, waking up dehydrated will be a poor start to your day. With this in mind, you also don't want to chug 32 oz. of water right before sleep, as this will likely cause you to wake up at some point in the night to relieve yourself. Ideally, you will be monitoring your hydration throughout the day, and just require a mild adjustment to achieve homeostasis.

The second piece is making sure you have gone to the bathroom before sleep. No one enjoys those dreams where you keep seeing toilets because your bladder is full. Avoid this unnecessary cause of awakening and make sure that you go to the bathroom right before you sleep every night.

Thirdly, try to take care of as much tomorrow stuff today. In other words, make sure you have cleaned, pressed clothing for work tomorrow. Make sure you have enough food for lunches or dinner. The more prepared you can be for tomorrow, the less likely your brain is to worry, and the better your sleep will be.

Lastly, make sure your phone is set to cause no interruptions other than your phone alarm. Even better, use an actual alarm clock, leaving your phone in fully silent mode. The jarring feeling that you experience as you are just dozing off into dreamland, only to be dinged awake by the sound of a text message, is infuriating. Make sure that once you decide it's time for bed, there will be no more disruptions.

There may be miscellaneous other activities that you need to perform prior to bed, such as: CPAP machine, retainer, applying special skin creams, earplugs, face mask, etc. These are also important as they will prevent your brain from worrying about them as you try to fall asleep, and they also set the stage for sleep, as your brain prefers routine and patterns to cue that it's bedtime.

My personal strategy is to create a checklist of the things I want in place before I sleep. By going through the checklist quickly before I go to bed, I make sure that I haven't forgotten anything, and this certainty actually leads to a better night's rest since my subconscious isn't stressed about something that I may have forgotten.

Below are some possible actions that you can start now to improve your sleep. The benefits will be pronounced and allow you to reap the rewards of high quality sleep immediately.

1. Stick to a routine. Doing the same thing each night will make it easier to fall asleep and stay asleep. Specifically, try to make your weeknights and your weekends as similar as possible. If you go to bed at 10:30 on Thursday, try to go to bed by 11pm on Friday.
2. Determine the ideal amount of time your body needs to sleep each night. Wake up without an alarm clock a few times on days that you don't have to work. Record how many hours you slept

each night and average them—this is generally how many hours of sleep your body needs to feel rested.

3. Avoid chemicals that disturb your natural sleep tendencies. No stimulants after noon, no alcohol within two hours of bedtime.

4. Make sure to go to the bathroom before you lie down.

5. Silence all notifications on your phone with the exception of the alarm.

6. Ensure adequate hydration status to avoid waking up with a desert mouth.

7. Avoid foods high in carbohydrates up to two hours of bedtime. Generally, try to avoid eating close to bedtime, but if you must eat something, foods with high protein disturb your sleep less than foods with high carbohydrates.

8. Use stimulants first thing in the morning to minimize sleep inertia.

9. If you need to take a nap, take one 15-minute nap around 2pm to ward off afternoon sleepiness.[11]

10. If having trouble falling asleep, use white noise, a sleep mask, or earplugs. If still ineffective, consider a different mattress.

11. Avoid bright lights and electronic screens 30 min. prior to bedtime.

Bill and Carol's Thoughts

Sleep had always been an issue for Carol, and occasionally for Bill. She would stay up at night thinking about everything she needed to do the next day, or get up early, just so her anxiety wouldn't interfere with her sleep any longer. She was very familiar with the effects of too little sleep, and recognized that if she only received four hours of sleep, though her body could make it through the next day, her mind was never quite right. This podcast finally broke down the scientific basis of sleep into its essential components, using simple analogies that made sense. Now she realized why it had been so hard for her to remember anything after having her first child: the lack of sleep with a newborn child negatively affects one's memory.

The action steps at the end of each podcast made deciding what to do next very simple. Obviously, they were doing some things correctly already. They didn't go out late on the weekends, so making their weekdays look like their weekends was pretty easy—although, sometimes they would watch SNL and push their usual bedtime back about an hour. The amount of time her body needed to sleep was probably 7.5 hours, though she thought waking up without an alarm clock the next couple of mornings would be a fun experiment.

While Carol would occasionally have decaf coffee after dinner, Bill would sometimes have an espresso. He would claim that it didn't affect his sleep, but Carol could tell that he didn't sleep as well on those nights. After listening to this, Bill decided that the espresso wasn't worth it, and would opt for a decaf espresso or skip it in the future. The same was true for his late-night whiskey. Bill decided that he would have his drinks earlier in the day or skip them to avoid damaging his sleep.

The part that talked about eating food close to bedtime would be a little more difficult—both Carol and Bill had long enjoyed their desserts. But hearing how high carbohydrate foods had a negative impact on sleep, they decided to start having their dessert earlier in the day, either with breakfast or lunch.

Giving up sweets was not an option, but changing when they were eaten seemed a fair compromise.

Bill found the bit about naps very enlightening. Originally he had assumed that naps should be an hour or two in length. After hearing the podcast, he thought that 15 minutes was almost not worth it, but that he'd give it a try. He did admit that he would often wake up from his afternoon naps feeling so groggy that it would take him until dinner before he felt fully alert again. Hopefully, these shorter naps would give him the physical pep he needed without the mental fogginess.

Carol paid close attention to the information about avoiding bright screens and using white noise to fall asleep, as this was her most difficult aspect of sleeping. She did use her cell phone right before bed, like most people, and knew that putting down the phone would be difficult. She decided that working on her book list at night would be a good move, and putting on a fan in the background could provide the white noise that she was looking for. She'd hold off on the face mask for the time being, and see how those small improvements helped.

References

1. Zager, Adriano, et al. "Effects of Acute and Chronic Sleep Loss on Immune Modulation of Rats." *American Journal of Physiology-Regulatory, Integrative and Comparative Physiology* 293.1 (2007): R504-R509.
2. Xie, Lulu, et al. "Sleep Drives Metabolite Clearance from the Adult Brain." *Science* 342.6156 (2013): 373-377.
3. Taheri, Shahrad, et al. "Short Sleep Duration is Associated with Reduced Leptin, Elevated Ghrelin, and Increased Body Mass Index." *PLoS Med* 1.3 (2004): e62.
4. Alhola, Paula, and Päivi Polo-Kantola. "Sleep Deprivation: Impact on Cognitive Performance." *Neuropsychiatric Disease and Treatment* 3.5 (2007): 553.
5. Hirshkowitz, Max, et al. "National Sleep Foundation's Sleep Time Duration Recommendations: Methodology and Results Summary." *Sleep Health* 1.1 (2015): 40-43.
6. Boutrel, Benjamin, and George F. Koob. "What Keeps Us Awake: the Neuropharmacology of Stimulants and Wakefulness-Promoting Medications." *Sleep-New York Then Westchester-* 27 (2004): 1181-1194.
7. Taheri, Shahrad, et al. "Short Sleep Duration is Associated with Reduced Leptin, Elevated Ghrelin, and Increased Body Mass Index." *PLoS Med* 1.3 (2004): e62.
8. Parmeggiani, Pier Luigi. *Systemic Homeostasis and Poikilostasis in Sleep*. London: Imperial College Press, 2011.
9. Tassi, Patricia, and Alain Muzet. "Sleep inertia." *Sleep Medicine Reviews* 4.4 (2000): 341-353.
10. Wertz, Adam T., et al. "Effects of Sleep Inertia on Cognition." *Jama* 295.2 (2006): 159-164.
11. Zaregarizi, Mohammad, et al. "Acute Changes in Cardiovascular Function During the Onset Period of Daytime Sleep: Comparison to Lying Awake and Standing." *Journal of Applied Physiology* 103.4 (2007): 1332-1338.

6 EATING

Bill noticed the improvements in his sleep right away. Ever since he had changed his naps, and avoided alcohol, carbohydrates and caffeine near bedtime, he was sleeping better than ever. He found that he had more energy in the morning, more willpower during the day, and felt like his mind was sharper than ever. Better yet, he noticed that his back pain had improved, and he had lost another pound over the week. He was beginning to really enjoy this health journey and noted that hadn't given up his favorite foods or subscribed to any fad diets either.

Carol had also noticed an improvement in how quickly she fell asleep. The lack of screen time before bed, coupled with the white noise, seemed to calm her down a bit quicker than before, and she was getting more sleep as a result. She even experimented with no alarm clock to see what her body needed, and it was nearly 7.5 hours exactly. With her improved sleep came improved energy levels and mental clarity, and she found that she was more productive throughout the day. She, too, had continued to lose an additional pound of weight, and was really starting to feel momentum building in her health journey.

Sixth Podcast

Portion Control

We're visual creatures. That is why moving advertisements on the corner of the computer screen catch our attention, and why strip clubs have been around for centuries. As humans, we make many of our decisions based on the visual information our brains receive. This strategy can be valuable when deciding on our home decor, but when applied to the nutritional requirements of our bodies, things go awry.

Here's the problem. The signals that we should be relying on to indicate fullness and satiety come from our stomach and gastrointestinal (or enteric) nervous system, not our eyes. If we rewind the tape of human history to a time before we put food onto plates and ate with silverware, food may not have been portioned out for us like it is today. Rather, we may have sat around a communal area and ate family style, eating as much as we needed until we felt full. Nowadays, however, the act of portioning out food determines the amount of food we eat to a larger degree than our internal feedback system of fullness and satiety.

So what is the solution? While it is not reasonable for every meal to be family style, and buying smaller plates and bowls sounds like an inconvenience, the real solution is to simply *slow down when we eat*. I have worked in restaurants for over a decade and have seen thousands of Americans eat meals. What I have noticed is just how quickly we scarf down our food without truly enjoying it. By slowing down, we will not only enjoy the food we eat more, savor the flavors and the aromas, and truly experience the full pleasure of eating, but we will allow time for our natural signals of fullness and satiety to reach our brain. As we slow down, our stomach and our enteric nervous system will signal to our brain that we are full, and to stop eating. This is the best way to control portion sizes in the long run. This is also a good strategy to control binge eating as well.[1]

So next time you wonder whether the size of the bowl or plate makes the difference, remember that the best thing you can do to decrease the amount of food you eat is to slow down and enjoy every bite; your stomach will tell your brain when you've had enough.

Eat Like an Omnivore

We're omnivores. That means we eat just about anything that doesn't kill us. It is also a major reason why we were able to evolve into this highly successful species. If we'd had a limited diet, we might have never been able to provide adequate nutrients to keep our calorie-hungry brain fueled every day.

But what does that mean for our diets today? Should we eat a paleo diet? A vegetarian diet? A pescetarian diet? A vegan diet? How do we know what is healthiest when nearly every month there is a new diet that claims to offer unparalleled health?

The truth is that there is no "perfect" diet. A diet

serves a function, and if you are an athlete living in Kenya, your diet should be drastically different from an Inuit living in the Arctic.

Regarding what each of us should eat, I am a fan of Michael Pollan's book, *In Defense of Food*, where he provides simple instructions: eat food, not too much, mostly plants.[2] Also, he advocates eating whole foods, prepared simply, and avoiding processed foods, especially ones containing a multitude of ingredients. Notice how he doesn't exclude whole parts of the food pyramid by deleting all meats, or all animals, or all grains.

Also important to keep in mind is that there are only three macronutrients: carbohydrates, lipids (or fats as we commonly refer to them), and proteins. While alcohol is routinely consumed and contains calories, it doesn't provide us with any essential nutrients and will be excluded in this discussion. At various times throughout history, society has shunned both fat and carbohydrates, with extreme diets that exclude an entire macronutrient cropping up to capitalize on this trend. The problem is that if we cut out carbohydrates, we must consume more fat and vice versa. Why? Because our body can only process a certain amount of protein before adverse effects occur. In general, humans need no more than 20% of their total calories from protein sources, meaning if you consume a 2500 calorie diet, then 500 calories, or 125 grams of protein would be the upper limit.[3] Consuming higher amounts of protein can damage your kidneys, liver, bones, and various other organs, as well as increasing your risk of certain cancers.[4] While the nutrition community is beginning to change their attitude towards fats as a healthier source of calories, we need to be mindful that cutting out a whole macronutrient category will leave us with an abundance of another. If I remove all carbs, then I am consuming 2000 calories of fat each day and 500 calories of protein. If I remove all fats, then I am consuming 2000 calories of carbs each day and 500 calories of protein. It is simple math that leads to startling results, and a thoroughly unbalanced diet.

The bottom line: eat whole foods in moderation, not indulging excessively in any one particular area. Don't cut out all meats, or all grains, or all anything. Rather, listen to your body and determine which foods work best for you and make you feel the healthiest. Remember that we have been omnivores for hundreds of thousands of years. Don't throw that evolutionary wisdom away on a fad diet and risk hurting your health.

Why Micro Is NOT the Answer

Science has done a great job of breaking complex things down to their smaller constituents. Whether it be examining cells under an electron microscope, or smashing protons together in a particle accelerator, science is always trying to find all the contributing parts of the whole.

Enter nutritional science of the twentieth century. Dietitians and nutritional scientists over the past 100 years have obsessed over finding every micronutrient in our foods and then calculating the proper amount required for each American, referred to as the Recommended Daily Allowance (RDA). As long as each person consumes the full amount of each micronutrient daily, then all of our nutritional needs will be met. It sounds simple enough, so where's the problem?

Taking a brief detour into the world of quantum physics may help explain the folly in this method of determining which foods to eat. Quantum physics is chiefly focused on particles, and much of the cutting edge research relies on detecting new particles using expensive particle accelerators. Yet the Newtonian laws of motion, the same laws that underlie the core of most introductory physics textbooks, may never have been deduced by examining quantum particles. There is, to date, no particle that is specifically responsible for gravity—or a graviton, as some refer to the hypothetical particle. Yet failing to apply gravity or the laws of motion, and exclusively using quantum physics, would have prevented much of our technological development of the twentieth century. While quantum physics does a better job of explaining what is happening on the particle level, it does a fairly poor job of explaining the principles involved in building a bridge.

Similarly, while nutritional science does a good job of explaining how each of these micronutrients is utilized by every cell in our body, it does a poor job at determining which foods are actually healthy or unhealthy. In order to determine that information, it is better to look at the entire piece of food, and not its micronutrients. It is becoming increasingly clear that we incorrectly villainized all saturated fats, making Americans pursue an anti-fat diet for several decades that has ultimately left us less healthy than if we had eaten more fat.[5] Saturated fat is much more complicated than we first thought, and discovering every facet of which type of fat is good or bad could take years. But what we do know is that if we focus on *foods*, then we can determine which foods are healthiest for us to eat. Focusing on micronutrients will only mislead us into anti-fat or anti-carb fads that will likely have the opposite effect of what we intended. Therefore, it is time that we stopped focusing on what percentage of saturated fat or how many grams of fiber we consume, and more on which foods we eat. It is time to stop focusing on the trees and observe the whole forest.

Timing Is Everything

Don't eat carbs. Don't eat fat. Don't eat meat. Fat makes you fat. Carbs make you fat. Meat makes you fat. The French paradox, the Mediterranean diet, the Inuit, the Maasai, the multitude of populations with diverse diets that all seem to be healthier than Americans following the newest diet trend. We've heard it all before, we've possibly tried it once or twice, but what we can all agree on is that we're thoroughly confused. Why are the French seemingly able to eat empty carbohydrates but don't suffer the same rates of diabetes and obesity as Americans? Why are the Inuit able to eat nearly 70% of their calories as fat, yet don't suffer from cardiovascular disease at anywhere near the rate that Americans do? How can a Mediterranean diet, of which the major component is grains, produce such a healthy population as compared to Americans?

The answer lies in timing. *When* you eat food is almost as important as *what* you eat. Here's the thing. Our bodies change throughout the day in terms of energy demands, hormone levels, and resting metabolic rate. Additionally, different activities use different energy forms such as glycogen (stored glucose) or adipose (stored fat), depending on the intensity of the activity. This means that eating a bagel in the morning is drastically different from eating a bagel before going to bed.

Here are the basics. First thing in the morning your body wants carbohydrates. You are waking up, your metabolism is ramping up, and your brain craves simple sugars to start all those neurons firing so you can get to work and focus. You will be up and about, moving around, and your body will utilize the majority of these carbohydrates as energy. Additionally, by having these carbohydrates early, you will be less likely to crave them later in the day. During lunch, your body wants a larger meal, one replete with fat and protein and some carbs. This is often the opposite of the American lunch, where we eat a light salad that doesn't fully satisfy us, leaving us starving come dinner, only to have us overeat at the worst possible time: night. We should eat a large meal at lunch, and if you drink alcohol, have the alcohol with lunch. Then, come dinner time, have a smaller meal, with a higher level of protein than either breakfast or lunch, and a lower level of carbohydrates. Avoid having simple carbohydrates or alcohol within two hours of going to bed.

Your body performs most of its repair and rebuilding while you sleep and will efficiently use late-night protein. But if you eat a sweet dessert right before dinner, the resulting insulin spike will turn nearly all of those carbs into adipose tissue (stored fat). Additionally, by drinking alcohol at night, you increase your insulin output as well, furthering fat deposition, as well as disturbing your REM sleep, making you less focused and mentally foggy the next day.

Bottom line: no single food group is bad or evil, but our bodies have different requirements depending on the time of day. Eat your carbs in the morning, your fat and alcohol at lunch, and your protein at night to maximize your satisfaction and your health.

The Power of Insulin

The Atkins Diet, the South Beach diet, the ketogenic diet, the glycemic diet, *Wheat Belly*—they are all leaning on the same principle: insulin makes you fat. This is pretty simple, and has been understood for decades by scientists. But putting it into practice often leads to extreme diets that are either unsustainable or end up being unhealthy through their reliance on processed foods and artificial sweeteners.

Insulin is a peptide hormone normally released by your pancreas in response to your blood sugar level. Insulin allows glucose to be taken up by cells, which then use it for fuel or convert it into fat. In healthy individuals, insulin levels rise after a meal, and within a couple hours insulin levels, along with blood sugar levels, have usually returned to baseline.[6] This process works well in healthy people, and creates the homeostasis for a constant blood sugar that our cells and tissues prefer.

In people with type I diabetes (insulin-dependent), their immune systems attack the cells in their pancreas that secrete insulin, making these individuals unable to regulate their blood sugar levels. Without insulin, these diabetics become very thin, unable to either access the sugar in their diet or convert those sugars to fat. As a result, diabetics without insulin are often hungry, have elevated blood sugar levels, and feel weak and fatigued. By injecting insulin, their cells can once again access these sugars and convert sugar to fat, allowing them to gain weight and regulate their blood sugars.

But what happens to healthy individuals if they continue to flood their bodies with very high levels of sugars that enter the bloodstream rapidly? The pancreas, sensing a massive rise in blood sugar, excretes a huge amount of insulin. This causes a rapid uptake of sugar into our cells. Since the amount of sugar exceeds the fuel requirements for these cells, much of the sugar is converted into fat, rather than being burned as fuel. Over time, the cells, being flooded with very high levels of insulin, become resistant to insulin levels. The cells require increasingly larger amounts of insulin to respond appropriately to the sugar levels. Eventually, the cells no longer uptake the sugars the way they are supposed to, leading to higher and higher levels of insulin, but now with paradoxically higher levels of sugars. At this point the person is pre diabetic and at risk for developing type II diabetes. If this continues without a quick lifestyle change, this person will soon require medication and eventually additional insulin to keep his blood sugar regulated. Of course, with additional insulin comes fat accumulation, and the cycle continues.

What should we do with this information then? Avoid all foods that trigger insulin release? Then we should be sure to lose weight, right? Yes and no. Yes, it is true that avoiding foods with high glycemic indexes (the glycemic index is a scale that indicates how much glucose is released into your blood over a fixed time after ingestion of a specific food) will decrease insulin release and result in weight loss. This is not a bad idea. The only problem is that the glycemic index is influenced by many factors besides just the food itself, such as how it was prepared, and what else is served with it. Obsessing about glycemic index is confusing and frustrating, and certainly not feasible for children or people with little patience. Instead, be mindful about foods with processed or refined starches, such as sugar, pasta, mashed potatoes and white bread. These foods tend to cause spikes in your insulin levels and do contribute to weight gain. Also, remember that our brain craves glucose and we love sugar, so don't expect to successfully cut all sugars out of your diet. Instead, focus on the timing of when you eat sugars, and try to have them early in the morning when you will be active, rather than right before bedtime when you will be sure to convert those sugars into fat.

Lastly, insulin is a powerful hormone, used for multiple processes such as growth and repair, not just for regulating blood sugar levels. Like everything, moderation is key, and avoiding all carbohydrates is a recipe for disaster, along with a rebound weight gain—the worst thing possible for achieving your ideal weight.

What you can do:

1. Slow down when you eat. You may want to set some small goals at first, such as only taking one bite every 30 seconds, until you are able to eat slowly more consistently.

2. Listen to your stomach for signals that you are full. Fullness does not come from your eyes, so listen to your stomach for that feeling of fullness and satiety.

3. Avoid the desire to "finish your plate" or empty the container when you've already eaten enough.

4. Try to eat family-style if possible, or at least take smaller portions initially, and only come back for seconds if you are still hungry.

5. Focus on choosing healthy *foods* rather than chasing after specific *nutrients*.

6. Choose whole foods over processed foods when available.

7. Choose a variety of foods, trying not to remove an entire category of the food pyramid.

8. Eat a balanced diet, meaning that if you had steak last night, try not to eat steak for a few nights at least. Too much of nearly anything can lead to adverse outcomes.

9. If you have the time or willpower, make your food at home as often as you can. This way, *you* control the amount of salt and processing in the food, not a company.

10. Embrace whole foods such as butter and lard over processed foods like margarine and hydrogenated oils. While butter may have higher levels of saturated fats, evidence has shown that the hydrogenated oils in margarine are more likely to contribute to coronary artery disease than natural sources of fat.[7]

11. Eat carbs early in the morning.

12. Eat more fat and alcohol at lunch, or early afternoon.

13. Eat more protein at dinner.

14. Avoid simple carbs and alcohol up to two hours before bed.

15. If drinking, choose wine over beer, as the amount of carbs is much lower in wine.

Bill and Carol's Thoughts

As Carol pondered the most recent podcast, she started to feel like she knew much of this information. In the recent weeks, she had already become more attuned to her body. She had slowed down her breathing, decreased her anxiety, become more mindful, and listened to her body for information about hydration status, energy levels, and aches and pains. The most recent information on slowing down while eating to listen to your natural signals of fullness seemed like common sense to her. This health thing was becoming easier each week, and the greatest part is that she hadn't had to spend a single dollar on any specialty food products.

Regarding the question of which diet was best, Carol had remembered seeing Michael Pollan on various interviews over the past decade, but had always viewed him as too extreme. After hearing the basics of the three macronutrients and how removing one, by definition, led to an unbalanced diet, she decided that perhaps there was more to this Michael Pollan guy than she had first thought. Since she was reading before bed at this point rather than using her phone, she decided to add his book to her list and give him a second shot.

Bill had always loved carbs and hearing that he shouldn't cut an entire category of foods out of his diet gave him huge relief. He loved his meat as well, and hearing that meat could be part of a balanced diet was also welcome news. Eating whole foods, some meat, a balance of whole grain unprocessed carbs and fresh veggies seemed like a very realistic diet. Additionally, learning that counting calories and obsessing about the number of saturated fat grams consumed each day was a waste of time, was truly liberating. Bill had grown weary of doctors, insufficiently trained in nutritional sciences, telling him how many grams of this or that food he could eat. He had seen eggs go from villain to hero more times than he could remember, and pork lard go from the worst fat possible, to a fairly healthy alternative to oil. Through this whole time he had felt frustrated with the lack of certainty and consistency from nutritional experts, and felt that they really knew less than they thought. Hearing vindication of his suspicions was refreshing, and allowed Bill to focus on foods that he grew up eating, foods that his mother and grandmother worked hard to prepare for him.

The part about timing had been touched upon in previous podcasts, but was clearly spelled out here. The whole French paradox thing made perfect sense. The French ate bread and croissants and pastries in the morning, yet their health was vastly superior to Americans. Armed with the knowledge of when to eat certain foods as well, he would be able to indulge in baked goods like croissants, without contributing to his belly fat in the process. The idea of having a glass of milk near bedtime made a lot of sense, since whole milk has a good amount of protein and fat. The recent trend towards skim milk and sugary foods directly before bedtime had been a setback to the nation's health. Similar to how the composition of breast milk changes during a feeding session to provide satiety to an infant, the diet consumed during the day should adjust to accommodate the energy demands of the body. Sleep was for rebuilding our cells, and therefore protein closer to bedtime was preferred. Simple sugars were the preferred energy source for our brain, so they would be most beneficial first thing in the morning. Relaxation and digestive powers were highest in the afternoon, and therefore this would be the ideal time for a large meal, replete with fat and protein. After hearing this, it seemed like common sense, but many Americans seemed to be doing it all wrong.

For Bill, the part about insulin and fat was far too real. During his visit six months ago, the doctor had told him that he was pre-diabetic. Bill knew what diabetes was (one of his friends had been diagnosed with it) and wasn't excited about the possibility of having to stick a needle into his stomach multiple times a day. Yet, he didn't want to cut out all sugars either. Hearing the science of what sugar and insulin actually did helped him realize what the problem was. A few changes to his diet such as swapping out the beer for wine, eating his sweets in the morning, and reducing the amount of pasta and rice on his plate were certainly realistic changes that would have substantial benefits. It was so relieving to hear someone talk about carbohydrates and sugar in a tone that didn't make Bill feel like an insolent child for wanting to eat them. Cutting back was doable, but eliminating them altogether just seemed crazy.

As for Carol, she had already been cooking more food at home. Now, she felt more pressure on her to buy healthy whole foods, and make them tasty to keep the momentum they both had created in the recent weeks. Luckily, she knew that, increasingly more grocery stores had fresh salad bars with slightly prepared foods that were minimally processed and not overly expensive. Breaking up her cooking nights with a meal from the salad bar would be a nice relief for her from the constant cooking, yet still adhere to the healthier food choices that they were committed to keeping.

References

1. Bello, Nicholas T., and Andras Hajnal. "Dopamine and Binge Eating Behaviors." *Pharmacology Biochemistry and Behavior* 97.1 (2010): 25-33.
2. Pollan, Michael. *In Defense of Food: An Eater's Manifesto.* Penguin, 2008.
3. Dietary Guidelines Advisory Committee. "Scientific Report of the 2015 Dietary Guidelines Advisory Committee." *Washington (DC): USDA and US Department of Health and Human Services* (2015).
4. Trichopoulou, A., et al. "Low-Carbohydrate–High-Protein Diet and Long-Term Survival in a General Population Cohort." *European Journal of Clinical Nutrition* 61.5 (2007): 575-581.
5. Siri-Tarino, Patty W., et al. "Saturated Fats Versus Polyunsaturated Fats Versus Carbohydrates for Cardiovascular Disease Prevention and Treatment." *Annual Review of Nutrition* 35 (2015): 517.
6. Melmed, Shlomo; Polonsky, Kenneth S; Larsen, P Reed; Kronenberg, Henry M. *Williams Textbook of Endocrinology 13th Edition.* Philadelphia: Elsevier, 2016. Print
7. Willett, W. C. "Dietary Fats and Coronary Heart Disease." *Journal of Internal Medicine* 272.1 (2012): 13-24.

7 THE WEIGHT LOSS INDUSTRY

The food podcast had contained a ton of information for both Carol and Bill. For the first time in many years, however, they both felt that they had a good grasp of what to eat. They had confidence that they understood what effect sugars could have on their weight if not controlled, but that they didn't have to cut anything out completely. They also realized that while making your own food does take more time, by staying home and controlling their exposure they weren't being tempted by processed garbage and high-calorie desserts. In fact, Carol really enjoyed spending more time at home with Bill, and Bill had re-engaged in cooking with her as well. They were both excited to test some of their newly learned recipes on their children next time they visited.

Seventh Podcast

The Trap of Weight Loss

Weight loss is easy—that's right, I said it. Setting a weight-loss goal, sticking to a specific diet for a specified amount of time, and losing a set amount of pounds is something that people have shown time and again is very achievable.[1] But keeping the weight off is nearly impossible.

So why do we continue to be seduced by companies whose sole allure is to help us lose weight?

The problem here is a difference between the means and the end. We all want good health, which is the end, but we become confused about the means to that end. We have been convinced that losing weight is the path to becoming healthy, but research has shown that simply isn't true. Not only is weight poorly correlated with health, but weight loss through diets is not sustainable, and worse, losing weight and regaining the weight may make you more susceptible to gaining weight in the future.[2]

But weight loss is sexy, it's seductive, and it's easy. It is objective, measurable, and immediately apparent within weeks of undertaking a program. It is addicting, and rewarding, and provides an injection of confidence when stepping outside. Weight loss is like a drug that we all love, but like a drug, eventually our body says "enough is enough," and the weight-loss high slows to a halt.

The solution for these companies is to take the discipline and willpower out of your hands by having you subscribe to their services indefinitely. By buying their food products or going to their meetings every week or month, you are caught in a perpetual fight to keep the pounds off, and they are in a position of making millions of dollars off your dependency.[3]

I don't want you to become dependent on another company for your weight loss, nor do I want you to be seduced by the siren song of weight loss at all. Rather, learn to *independently* manage your health, and focus on becoming truly healthy in the long run, not on the short-term allure of weight loss.

Diets and Cognitive Dissonance

Cognitive dissonance: the state of having inconsistent thoughts, beliefs, or attitudes, especially as relating to behavioral decisions and attitude change. Why did I just define that? Because when we delve into the world of diets, it is around every corner... let me explain.

When we undertake to follow a diet, let's say a diet with less than 50 grams of carbohydrates per day, we are consciously deciding that we will stick to this diet, and that our behaviors will align with our goals. At first, everything goes well, and the pounds start coming off. Then, we have our first moment of weakness. It's Bob's birthday, and there's delicious chocolate cake, and the whole staff is eating it, so why not just have one piece—you'll make up for it the next day? Then BOOM! It hits you, the awful feeling that ensues, which forces us to make a decision.

Your brain begins an inner dialogue with itself.

Ideal self: "Wait, did you just eat a piece of cake, and ruin the diet that you've been following so faithfully for the past two weeks?"

Realistic self: "Yes, but it was only once in the past

two weeks, and I'll make up for it tomorrow."

Ideal self: "But if you've already broken the diet today, then it doesn't really matter what else you eat today, you should just call this day a wash and enjoy yourself."

Realistic self: "I suppose you're right. I mean, if I couldn't even stick to this diet plan, then I'm sort of a failure. I should just give up today, and we'll start over again tomorrow, and then I promise I'll stick to the diet."

And on, and on...

Regardless of what *your* inner dialogue sounds like, the ultimate goal of your brain is to reduce or eliminate this cognitive dissonance, which can be very painful and uncomfortable. We will do anything to make sure that our behavior (our adherence to our diet) align with our belief (that we can follow this diet). When our behavior and our belief are not aligned, we are in a state of cognitive dissonance, and we struggle to escape from the awful feeling.

Ultimately, reality always wins, and we *will* break the diet, because adhering to a strict diet devoid of an entire macronutrient is not only unrealistic, it's also unsustainable for a lifetime. The only way to avoid the pain of cognitive dissonance is to avoid diets altogether and live your life with the flexibility and realism that accompanies being human in a world with birthday cake.

Diets and External Cues

Our bodies are speaking to us constantly. As mentioned previously, we need to listen to our bodies to determine the effects of our actions. Eat a greasy bacon double cheeseburger, and notice how your body feels heavy and slow later in the day. Your body wants to communicate with you so that you may make the best decisions for your health every day.

Diets, on the other hand, teach us to ignore what our body is saying to us. Instead, they turn our attention to external cues like the amount of points we've accumulated, how many calories we've consumed, or portion sizes, rather than relying on our own body's feedback of feeling full and satiated.[4] Over time, we begin to ignore our body, shutting out the useful information it provides us, and becoming oblivious to its messages. We obsess about the external cues, forgetting that our body has anything to say at all.

Eventually, we find ourselves utterly dependent on these external cues. Frantically counting points, or calories, or other inane details, we no longer notice if we are hungry, or full, or frankly if we even feel healthy. We have surrendered ourselves to the newest external scheme to control our diet and our health, and in the process have become unable to control our behaviors without these crazy calculations and algorithms present.

Eating should not be a math problem. Our bodies should not be ignored. We have intricately, beautifully designed bodies that will provide us with all the necessary information to independently manage our weight and eat healthily... we just need to break free from the external cues and listen to our bodies once again.

A List of behaviors to help you maintain your ideal weight:

1. Never *diet*—**period.**
2. Avoid all schemes, algorithms, points-based systems, or any other type of program that focuses on external cues rather than internal cues to guide your eating decisions.
3. Focus on all of the factors that lead to health such as sleep, stress, etc., and not just on weight. Excess weight is a *symptom* of an unhealthy life, not the *problem*.
4. Listen to your body to guide you in deciding what foods to eat, when to eat, and how much to eat. We have all the tools to allow us to manage our food intake ourselves.
5. Mind your mental well-being. Eating and overeating is often a habit that develops in response to issues occurring at the psychological level. Address your psychological demons and the desire to overeat will diminish.
6. Stop comparing your weight to anyone else's. Everyone has different body types and different levels of hormones that contribute to our beautiful diversity. Your ideal weight is not determined by someone else, but by you alone.

Bill and Carol's Thoughts

By now, these podcasts were almost echoing Carol and Bill's lives, rather than being as prescriptive and difficult as they had first imagined. While it was certainly true that Carol used to battle with weight loss and had subscribed to numerous weight loss fads and diets, she found that she no longer thought about weight loss as a goal in itself. Rather, she realized that health was the goal, and that in the process of living a healthy life, she would achieve her ideal weight.

Regarding her previous diet fads, she had subscribed to Weight Watchers, Atkins, Paleo, Low-fat, Essential Oils and the smoothie diet, to name a few. Despite losing weight on each diet, she inevitably gained it all back, and sometimes more, within a couple years of starting each one. The podcast finally shed light on the truth that these companies were more interested in generating consumer dependency and massive profits than they were in improving people's lives. It made sense why so many companies promoted this same pattern of dependency on a specific product or plan, since it was so profitable. This podcast, which simply offered free advice, made only a small amount of profit from the limited advertising. Clearly, that was not the kind of profit that large corporations wanted.

The part about cognitive dissonance resonated soundly with Carol. She clearly remembered numerous occasions when she would break one of her diets, and then feel awful immediately afterwards. Yet instead of forgiving herself for being human and working harder to avoid the same mistake, her brain would begin devising rules about why it was okay for her to break the diet today, or this week. Soon, her brain would have this elaborate inner dialogue, justifying why eating that second piece of cake was okay, and that she'd make up for it tomorrow by being stricter. In the end, Carol always ended up feeling like a failure with these unrealistic diets, and she hated herself for it. A strict diet sets you up to feel miserable, rather than creating a mindset of living healthfully while acknowledging that birthdays happen.

Bill agreed with the part about losing touch with

our bodies' signals, and relying on external cues. He, too, had felt frustrated by Carol's previous diets that required her to count calories, tally points, or prepare very specific foods a certain way. He had felt that it was silly to ignore the signals that every person's stomach provided, telling them that they were full. He had noticed, especially since he had been breathing more slowly and avoiding food late at night, how full he felt 30 minutes after eating. Now that he was having larger lunches, he found that he wasn't very hungry at dinner, and a small meal was more than enough to satisfy him until bedtime.

The bottom line is that our bodies are far smarter than any algorithm or point scheme that some profit-hungry corporation has created. By ignoring our bodies, we are merely ignoring the wisdom that has guided us for thousands of years.

References

1. Jeffery, Robert W., et al. "Long-Term Maintenance of Weight Loss: Current Status." *Health Psychology* 19.1S (2000): 5.
2. Zwaan, Martina, Stefan Engeli, and Astrid Müller. "Temperamental Factors in Severe Weight Cycling. A Cross-Sectional Study." *Appetite* 91 (2015): 336-342.
3. Staff, ABC News. "100 Million Dieters, $20 Billion: The Weight-Loss Industry by the Numbers." *ABC News*. ABC News, 8 May 2012.
4. Web. 17 Aug. 2016. "Introducing Beyond the Scale." *Weight Watchers: Our Approach*. Weight Watchers, n.d. Web. 17 Aug. 2016.

8 ACTIVITIES AND MOVEMENT

Despite not focusing on weight loss at all, Bill and Carol had each lost over five pounds in the last six weeks. While not very fast, it was sustainable, and the wonderful part was that they didn't feel like they were depriving themselves of anything in the process. In fact, since Bill had been doing his back exercises more consistently, and since he was sleeping better, he was now doing much more work around the house than before. He had even pulled out his old push mower instead of his ride-on lawn mower just to get the extra exercise. This new lifestyle never felt like a diet or a trick, but rather simply a better way to live that made him feel better as well.

Eighth Podcast

Posture, Gravity and the Tin Man

Gravity is waging a silent war against our joints every day. Each day it pulls down upon us, slowly shortening us, squeezing our vertebral discs, and gradually deforming our appearances. The result of this war is posture, or the position of the body when in a relaxed state, without excessive use of muscular force. If asked to stand for ten minutes, your body will eventually relax into its posture, providing a clear indication of which side is winning in the war between gravity and your joints.

In addition to gravity's effects on our joints, there is also time. Time acts on our joints like it does on the Tin Man from The Wizard of Oz: it dries them out until they become rigid. When we are young, we have lots of fluid in our joints, and they move easily, with full range of motion. As we age, our range of motion diminishes, and we notice that our joints become stiffer, similar to the Tin Man rusting.[1] If not moved for a few days, our joints may almost feel like rusted metal: stiff and resistant to all motion. This is why it is so important to move around every day and maintain your full range of motion for as long as possible.

The good news is that we have some control over this battle. We can't change gravity's effects (aside from going into space), and we can't slow down time (at least not yet), but we can decide how quickly our joints will rust (dry out), and in what position we will be in when it happens.

We are just like the Tin Man, who, if he stopped moving, would get stuck and need oil to move again. But if he had kept moving, he might not have needed any oil in the first place. So that's our first goal, to move our joints every day. I'm not talking about boring stretches for 30 minutes, but rather just moving our joints through their entire range. Running, jumping, dancing, and yard work: these are all activities that will do the trick.

The second goal is to pick the best position to be stuck in as our joints stiffen. In other words, the position in which we sit, stand, and even sleep will eventually be the position in which our joints remain. We have all seen older individuals whose heads are so low that they are struggling just to see in front of them. This did not take place overnight, but rather over decades. It was by keeping their head forward for months and years that eventually led to their spine stiffening in that position. At that point, it is too late to reposition their head directly between their shoulders, but if you act now to maintain good posture, you can prevent this fate for yourself.

The only things preventing you from having the posture and flexibility you want are the barriers. They include muscle weakness, muscle resistance, joint resistance, and nerve resistance.[2,3] As your posture becomes fixed, these three tissues reset their length and resist changes to it. They can be changed by actively stretching, which takes deliberate effort and time, as they will not reset on their own. Weakness in key muscles will also prevent you from maintaining proper posture. For information on how to best stretch these tissues and strengthen the key muscles to achieve certain postural goals, it is best to seek the advice of professionals, such as physical therapists, who will improve your efficiency and safety in these activities.

So now you know who the players are in this battle. They are gravity and time versus your joints, with your muscles and nerves playing a secondary role. By maintaining correct posture and keeping your joints moving, you can prevent having forward head position as you age, and while your flexibility will inevitably decline, you can still have the profile of a person much younger than you.

Exercise and Dogs

Greyhounds are bred to run; it's what they do. But ask a Corgi to run like that and it'll probably give up after 200 feet. A Border Collie will be happy to herd the flock all day with endless energy, but a Basset Hound would prefer to lounge.

Humans are like dogs—we are not all born to run. We have different body styles, different genetic makeups, and different proclivities for specific activities. The broad shoulders and general strength of a large Norwegian man make him ill-suited to running long distances. Likewise, the lithe but muscular bodies of the runners from Kenya and Ethiopia are not designed for raw strength, but rather are perfectly suited for running long distances.

I propose that we first replace the word "exercise" with activity, and secondly, stop focusing on which type of activity we do. We need to recognize that each person may be more suited to one activity over another, and that both can be the ideal form of physical exertion for that individual. The important element here is that we find an activity that we enjoy and perform it regularly. Whether it's running, cutting wood, or gardening, movement is what matters. As long as we are elevating our heart rate to some degree, moving our joints, and breaking a sweat, it will be beneficial.[4] The degree to which we enjoy what we're doing, however, will determine our success in that activity far more than anything else.

So let's stop trying to fit our body to the activity and instead find an activity that fits our body.

When Unplugging Gives You a Charge

The advent of electricity has changed daily life dramatically. We use washing machines instead of hand washing clothes, ride-on lawn mowers in place of push mowers, and the plethora of power tools available to even the most novice of craftsmen is staggering.

Yet, ignoring the saved time and physical effort for a moment, what have we lost by shifting to a world where electricity does the work that manpower used to?

What we've lost is the opportunity to perform meaningful activity that is both beneficial to our health as well as satisfying and enjoyable. You see, with most modern inventions we have removed the physical human component needed to perform the work, leaving us with organized exercise as the only logical way to acquire sufficient activity for health. The boredom and unsatisfying nature of running on a treadmill, or picking weights up just to put them down, however, is undeniable. If exercising was as interesting as we wished it was, we wouldn't have any trouble maintaining our ideal weight in the first place.

But what if we unplugged for a moment, and chose to perform the work that electricity now does for us? What if we decided to chop our own wood with an actual axe, and use our fireplace? What if we decided to clean our clothes occasionally on an old-fashioned washboard? What if we made fine wood products using saws and sandpaper rather than power tools? The result, rather than boredom, might be satisfaction from purposeful activity and a job well done. The ultimate result too, would be a greener earth, where humans no longer run in place on treadmills, but rather perform a multitude of activities that have meaning and produce usable products in an environmentally sustainable way.

What Does Core Really Mean?

We've all heard that we need to work on our core, but do we really know what that means?

Imagine a thin tree, swaying in the wind. The tree is weak, and easily bent by the strong winds. Over time, the tree will bend so far that it may break. In order to prevent this, we often build tree supports or tree cables, which provide support to the weak trunk.

In this analogy the tree trunk is our spine. By design, our spine is fairly weak and wobbly. It only stays upright due to the myriad muscles and ligaments around it. Our muscles in this analogy are the tree supports, or cables, that keep the tree from bending and breaking. By strengthening the muscles that connect to the spine, we can provide support to this inherently flimsy part of our skeleton and prevent injuries down the line. Simply put, our core is the collection of muscles that directly or indirectly connect to the spine and help to provide support against outside forces.

Continuing this analogy, imagine a thin tree with huge branches. Every gust of wind now pulls that tree harder than before due to the branches catching the wind. A person with huge arms is capable of generating massive forces, but if under his shirt he has a weak core, then he is at increased risk of injuring his back. The stronger your branches (arms) are, the stronger your core should be to help prevent injury. Therefore, next time you want to focus on building those biceps or shoulders, make sure to include some core exercises to keep your back healthy in the long run.

A list of activities that can replace some of your routine exercises:

1. Chop wood with an axe for use in your fireplace or wood-burning stove.
2. Make things out of wood using hand tools such as a saw, sandpaper, and a hammer and nails.
3. Wash dishes by hand.
4. Dry clothes on a clothesline.
5. Cook and bake at home.
6. Knead bread by hand.
7. Have animals that you take for walks and/or groom regularly.
8. Make ice cream using an old-fashioned ice cream maker.
9. Make butter using a butter churner.
10. Mow the lawn using an old-fashioned push-mower that simply requires sharpening of the blades.
11. Rake the yard rather than use a leaf blower.
12. Do landscaping around the house.
13. Plant trees and other plants.
14. Go fishing or hunting for dinner.
15. Tend a garden.
16. Start a compost pile.
17. Help friends move.
18. Help friends or neighbors with work around the house or yard.

Bill and Carol's Thoughts

What amazed Carol was that it had taken eight podcasts before exercise was directly discussed. Most health companies touted either heavy exercise or severe dietary changes in order to achieve health goals. Yet this podcast had waited several weeks before even mentioning exercise. Now that it had discussed exercise, it was so brief and simple that Carol was left wondering why huge books and complicated exercise programs had been written on a subject that at its core seemed so simple.

Bill had been nagged by his family and doctors alike about his posture for years. Working in a wine store, he had spent hours at the computer, updating inventory and ordering various products. That fixed position had taken a toll on him and his spine certainly wasn't erect as it could be. He hadn't really focused on posture, since his back pain occupied more of his attention, but since he was already seeing a physical therapist for his back, he figured that it couldn't hurt to ask his therapist for some exercises to address his posture. In the meantime, Bill knew that he could start modifying his computer setup and even his driving position to make sure that he spent the majority of his time in a better position. The idea of the Tin Man rusting with a forward head position gave him some serious concerns, and he didn't want that future for himself.

Meanwhile, the notion of just doing activities that match with your body style seemed like good common sense. Despite this logic, Carol could remember many of her friends telling her that this sport or that exercise was the "best" one to lose weight, or the "best" one for cardiovascular health. Running had never appealed to Carol, and at this point in her life, it might hurt her knees. Knowing that whether she decided to run or kayak did not matter—and that what mattered most was whether she enjoyed the activity—was a relief.

The part about unplugging to go back to traditional forms of movement appealed to Bill and Carol both. Bill had already gone back to his push mower for the exercise, and now he would do some edging and hedging with his older tools as well. Woodworking used to be one of Bill's hobbies as well, but he had never thought of it as an alternative to exercise. Now armed with this new perspective, he was eager to do yard work and help his neighbors with yard work, knowing that it would count as his exercise for the day. Carol, too, had enjoyed her time working on her sister's farm in the past. Now, she would try to spend more time on the farm, where the planting, tending, and harvesting would be great exercise for her, without the boring repetition of running or using the elliptical machine at the gym. By using their creativity and imagination, they were confident that they could find ways to exercise that were also productive, and that didn't feel repetitive and boring either.

The information on core was also very helpful for Bill. Despite having several meetings with doctors and physical therapists, he had never truly known what "core" meant. After listening to the podcast it finally made sense to him. He now understood why he needed to perform these "silly" exercises using muscles he couldn't see in order to protect his back. But, more importantly, he realized how many activities around the house could strengthen his core and be satisfying as well. While the exercises the physical therapist gave him were good when he was in pain, now that he was feeling better he sought to challenge himself with more substantial exercises such as chopping wood with an ax, or edging the driveway.

References

1. Boone, Donna C., and Stanley P. Azen. "Normal Range of Motion of Joints in Male Subjects." *J Bone & Joint Surgery Am* 61.5 (1979): 756-759.
2. Norris, Christopher M. "Spinal stabilisation: 2. Limiting Factors to End-Range Motion in the Lumbar Spine." *Physiotherapy* 81.2 (1995): 64-72.
3. Wright, Thomas W., et al. "Ulnar Nerve Excursion and Strain at the Elbow and Wrist Associated with Upper Extremity Motion." *The Journal of Hand Surgery* 26.4 (2001): 655-662.
4. American College of Sports Medicine. *ACSM's Guidelines for Exercise Testing and Prescription*. Lippincott Williams & Wilkins, 2013.

9 DISEASE

Over the next week Carol was surprised at how much work Bill did around the house. Rather than putting off yard work, it seemed like Bill was actively looking for new projects. Better still was that with the increased activity, Bill was sleeping even better, giving him more energy and making him more efficient during the day. Carol, too, had spent more time gardening, and started using a clothesline for her laundry when it was sunny out, rather than the dryer. While the goal was still health, it was fun for Carol to find ways to use less energy as they increased their activity levels too.

Ninth Podcast

The Lifestyle Diseases

A cure for cancer. An end to heart disease. The eradication of diabetes. Wouldn't it be wonderful if we could achieve all of these things in our lifetime?

The truth is that we already have the solution to all of these problems—we just have to look within ourselves, rather than to the healthcare system.

When looking at the top 10 causes of death in America, what becomes apparent is that they are largely lifestyle diseases.[1] In other words, the *way* that we live our lives determines to a large extent whether we will develop diabetes, cancer, or heart disease. How do we know this? By studying indigenous groups of people before the advent of industrialization, we can observe the natural rates of these diseases without modern Western influence.

Oft-cited groups of people that were largely devoid of these lifestyle diseases included the people of Okinawa, Sardinia, the Inuit and the Maasai. These people had virtually zero rates of heart disease, stroke, cancer and diabetes. All of their diets differed greatly, but some aspects of their lifestyles remained consistent. These people generally had a strong sense of community, often with a religious or spiritual component uniting them. Nearly all of the people were active their entire life, with even the elder women performing gardening and other tasks in their final years. They ate largely unprocessed, whole foods that were seasonally available, with limited curing, drying, or pickling as needed. In short, they led a simple, active life full of good food and good company.[2]

So the bottom line is that while we may feel that these lifestyle diseases are inevitable when we look around at our fellow Americans, it is actually possible to live a life free from these diseases by following a fairly simple but healthy path. The good news is that we don't have to wait for the scientists to come up with the cure… we already have it.

Skin Health and Chameleons

We are like chameleons. True, our skin doesn't change from green to blue, but our skin does change from peach to pink, to red, depending on various external factors. Our skin is the canvas of our body, representing minute-to-minute changes of what's going on beneath the surface. By learning what factors affect our skin, we can come closer to having that Maybelline complexion we so desire.

Sunlight, or more specifically ultraviolet radiation, is the single largest factor in our skin health. Ultraviolet rays damage our skin cells, including the DNA contained in those cells. This damage accumulates over months and years to accelerate the aging process, leaving increased wrinkles and decreased elasticity in its wake. The damage to the DNA in the basal layer of our dermis can contribute to cancerous cells, such as basal cell carcinoma. Most dermatologists agree that a daily application of sunscreen with moisturizer, applied to exposed body parts, especially the face and neck, is the best way to protect yourself against the ravaging effects of sunlight. While a tanned complexion is considered highly desirable by many people, what is certainly not desirable is a face full of wrinkles and sagging skin later in life as a result of not respecting the power of the sun. Remember, sunlight contains immense energy, and when directed towards our skin, the damage is undeniable. Protect your skin from this destructive energy and stay looking healthier than your similarly-aged peers.

Stress is probably the second most important factor in our skin health. While not 100% within our control, we can reduce our stress by slowing down our breathing. As you have already read in the chapter on stress, breathing and stress levels are closely related.

Diet and nutrition are of great importance to our skin health. Most significantly, sugars and other simple starches can wreak havoc on our skin, leading to acne, excess oil production, and inflammation. Certain high-fat foods can also irritate our skin, so keeping a balanced diet is essential for that blemish-free complexion.

Sleep. It seems to crop up everywhere and affect every system in our body. When we lose sleep, cortisol levels rise, and that is bad news for our skin. Cortisol can weaken the skin, increasing the chance of developing stretch marks, and worse, increasing our risk of skin infections. Reread the sleep chapter if this is still a problem for you.

Alcohol. While not harmful in low quantities (one to three drinks, depending on body weight), excess alcohol consumption will harm your skin through the three means listed above. Alcohol disrupts your sleep, leads to rebound stress, and also increases your blood sugar levels, which has a 1-2-3 punch on your skin health.

In summary, your skin is sensitive to everything going on inside and outside of your body, letting the world know if you've been up late drinking and eating sugary foods. By taking control of the major health behaviors in your life, your skin will soon reflect the healthy body inside, and reward you with a smooth, unblemished complexion.

Chronic Pain and Low Back Pain

Nearly every person will experience some type of low back pain in their lifetime.[3] Even more people will experience some type of chronic pain, which is pain that lasts for six weeks or longer. A large percentage of primary care physician visits are for low back pain or related chronic pain. The money spent on treating these problems is simply staggering.

So let's briefly review spinal anatomy and our nervous system to understand why this problem plagues so many people, and what you can do about it. The spine is a collection of vertebrae, or pieces of bone, supported by cartilaginous discs which contain a gel-like substance inside. Surrounding each disc is a crisscross arrangement of tough fibrous tissue that holds each disc firmly in place. Back injuries may take many forms, but commonly a disc injury is involved. What does not occur, however, is a disc "popping out". Rather, some of the fibrous tissue surrounding the disc tears, with the result being either a small rupture in the disc integrity, or sometimes an actual displacement of the gel-like substance outside of the disc. While these injuries are certainly painful and absolutely debilitating, they are usually not the life-sentence we think they are. The notion that you "slipped a disc" back in high school and it is still causing your pain 30 years later is simply incorrect.

So, with spinal anatomy covered, what role does the nervous system play in this annoying problem of back pain? Surrounding the vertebrae and discs are spinal nerves. These nerves are sensitive to pressure, chemicals, and alterations in blood flow, like most tissues. When a back injury occurs, these nerves may be injured, causing symptoms such as numbness, tingling, or shooting pain down the distribution of these nerves. This nerve damage may be temporary or permanent, but in most cases it is temporary. The few cases where the nerve damage may lead to lasting damage are where quick surgical intervention is advised. The good and the bad thing about our nervous system, however, is that it adapts. One adaptation that is not helpful is that certain chronic pains may alter the sensitivity of the nervous system. This means that particular stimuli such as pressure or temperature changes that previously did not cause pain may now cause pain after the injury.

While this is certainly bad news, the story isn't all negative. The good news is that our mood, stress and overall lifestyle can have a significant effect on whether our pain becomes disabling and chronic, or annoying and tolerable. By following a healthy lifestyle with movement, good sleep, low stress and healthy food, you can minimize the impact of back injuries and decrease the likelihood that you will become a victim of debilitating chronic pain yourself.

Actions you can take to minimize the risk of developing chronic pain:

1. Treat your pain quickly. Take ibuprofen or acetaminophen the day of the injury, and ice the area as well. The quicker you address the pain, the less likely it will develop into chronic pain.[4]
2. Keep moving. Our first instinct is to avoid activities that cause pain, for fear of producing greater damage. While you certainly will want to avoid specific movements that trigger intense pain,

you must try to keep moving and perform your daily routine as closely as possible. Taking weeks and months of time off from work has been shown to greatly increase the risk of developing chronic pain.[5]

3. Let go of the anatomy trap. This trap refers to the obsession some people develop about finding something on an X-ray or MRI that will correspond to their symptoms. The nervous system is pliable and may undergo changes in its sensitivity that are not visible on imaging. Recognize that not every source of pain has an anatomical location and that surgery is unlikely to be the answer for chronic pain.

4. Keep your stress levels low. Stress and anxiety have been shown to increase the rating of perceived pain.[6] Use the slow breathing strategy found earlier in the book to achieve this.

5. Get adequate, quality sleep.[7]

6. Use opioid-based pain medication as a last resort only. Research has shown that use of opioids may actually increase and prolong our pain experience.[8]

Immune System

Let's take this extremely complicated system and try to simplify it down to a few paragraphs, and then distill out what you can do to maximize its performance in your life. The immune system is sort of like the TSA at the airport. Its job is to scan and screen individuals (potential pathogens) who may be at risk to the plane (the organism). To be efficient it cannot screen every individual, but must make some quick judgments to ensure timely processing. Like our immune system, the TSA is prone to making mistakes, and is sometimes understaffed, causing certain dangerous individuals to infect the plane.

The more exposure to various "pathogens" the TSA encounters throughout their work schedule, the better they become at recognizing and disposing of these individuals. Similarly, the more exposure to bacteria and dirt, such as occurs when living on a farm, the stronger and more robust your immune system will be. Likewise, the more exposure your immune system has to pathogens at an early age, the more discriminating it will be against pathogens that are not real threats to your body, such as dust particles, etc. In this sense, your immune system learns to discriminate and to avoid attacking harmless offenders.

Additionally, the scrutiny that the TSA applies to each passenger is dependent on the current threat level. If there is a higher than normal suspicion of a terrorist in the building, they will begin screening more individuals and may be more aggressive with their dispositions of suspected terrorists. Similarly, the body's threat level may be adjusted depending on the environmental circumstances, such as one's diet, stress levels, activity levels, and amount of sleep the night before. When the threat level is increased, the body will attack more foreign invaders and mount a larger immune response.

To summarize, our body's immune system has to balance efficiency with comprehensiveness. It learns over time to be more efficient and more discriminatory in deciding which invaders are a threat (reacting differently to Salmonella as opposed to harmless dust particles). It can be ramped up to be more aggressive and more robust, or ramped down to be milder.

One obvious way in which we can ramp down our immune system, to the detriment of our health, is by failing to acquire sufficient high quality sleep. The physiology is quite simple. As we become sleep deprived our cortisol levels rise.[9] Cortisol is the major immunosuppressant hormone, or master switch, that largely determines the "threat level" of our immune system. As this hormone rises and remains elevated for prolonged periods of time, our body's immune system becomes lazy, in a sense, allowing little viruses that cause the common cold to infect us, when normally it would protect us.[10] The result is that a few nights of burning the candle at both ends will often lead to a cold.

Another way in which our behaviors affect our immune system is in our intestinal flora. The food that we eat has a significant impact on the threat level of our immune system. Americans tend to have a high amount of omega-6 fatty acids in their diet, especially compared to the levels of omega-3 fatty acids. The high levels of omega-6 fatty acids increase the threat level in our gut, causing our immune system to become aggressive and less discriminate. The result is an inflamed gut, with the host of symptoms such as bloating, cramping and gas that we often call irritable bowel syndrome.[11,12]

There are numerous other ways in which our behavior has direct effects on our immune system. Below is a list of actions you can take to ensure that your immune system is operating optimally:

1. Get quality sleep nightly.
2. Keep stress levels low.

3. Eat a healthy, balanced diet full of nutrient-rich plants, and low in refined starches and sugars.
4. Consume adequate levels of omega-3 fatty acids (fish oils) and moderate to low levels of omega-6 fatty acids (polyunsaturated oils like corn and soybean oil).
5. Be active, but not too active. Extreme exertion, like running a marathon, actually weakens your immune system for a few days.
6. Avoid binge-drinking episodes (more than four drinks in any one period).

Bill and Carol's Thoughts

While hearing a podcast about disease when you're trying to become healthier might have seemed a little negative, Carol appreciated the frank way in which it discussed issues like cancer and diabetes. The truth was that everyone would die of something, but we all hoped that it would be quick and painless. Watching her friends go through cancer and diabetes had scared her enough to take any precaution possible to avoid these same fates for herself. Hearing that avoiding cancer might be a matter of living a healthy lifestyle gave her a sense of control, and helped her avoid the feeling of helplessness that often led to depression. She had heard about the people of Okinawa before, but she wasn't aware that other cultures were largely devoid of diseases like cancer and heart disease as well.

The bit on skin health made perfect sense to Carol. Having struggled with the fickle nature of psoriasis, it was helpful to have someone summarize the way the skin responded to every external input like a chameleon. Carol had noticed, since embarking on this health journey, that her skin was much improved, and her psoriasis hadn't flared up recently. Reminding herself that her outside skin would reflect her inner health gave her further motivation to stay committed to her new lifestyle.

Bill was almost angry after hearing about back pain and chronic pain. He wondered why his physical therapist and especially his doctor hadn't explained these factors to him the way the podcast had. After learning how plastic the nervous system was, and how often the anatomy does not correspond with what was felt, he realized that he had more control over his back pain than he had originally thought. While it was true that Bill had injured his back on a few specific occasions while moving heavy wine cases, he remembered healing from each of those injuries individually. Bill had long believed that those injuries were still the source of his pain, due to some permanent disc displacement that couldn't be fixed. Now, he realized that it wasn't a disc displacement or some gross anatomical deformity that was causing his prolonged back pain, but rather his nervous system had become predisposed to causing him pain, almost as if it had learned to warn him of pain sooner than before.

With the information from the podcast, Bill could focus on those factors that would predispose his nervous system to cause him pain, or focus on activities and habits that would minimize his pain. Knowing that lack of sleep could increase his pain gave him more reason to respect the power of sleep. Learning that attacking new pains quickly with pain medication and ice was better than enduring it for days was also revelatory. It was refreshing to realize that Bill had much more control over his pain levels than he had previously believed, and this empowered him. Rather than focusing on anatomy and MRI reports, he could now focus on living a healthy life and managing his stress levels.

Armed with this new knowledge about disease and the immune system, Carol and Bill felt more prepared for the later years of their lives. They understood that their actions, and more specifically their health habits, were largely responsible for whether they'd acquire cancer, have a psoriasis flare-up, or get sick. This put their longevity squarely in their hands, rather than down to bad luck or chance. The future was looking brighter than ever.

References

1. Datz, T. "Smoking, High Blood Pressure and Being Overweight Top Three Preventable Causes of Death in the US." *Harvard School of Public Health* (2009).
2. Santrock, John (2008). "Physical Development and Biological Aging". In Mike Ryan, Michael J. Sugarman, Maureen Spada, and Emily Pecora (eds.): *A Topical Approach to Life-Span Development* (pp. 129-132). New York: McGraw-Hill Companies, Inc.
3. Vinod Malhotra; Yao, Fun-Sun F.; Fontes, Manuel da Costa (2011). *Yao and Artusio's Anesthesiology: Problem-Oriented Patient Management.* Hagerstwon, MD: Lippincott Williams & Wilkins. pp. Chapter 49. ISBN 1-4511-0265-8.
4. Fassoulaki, Argyro, et al. "Multimodal Analgesia with Gabapentin and Local Anesthetics Prevents Acute and Chronic Pain after Breast Surgery for Cancer." *Anesthesia & Analgesia* 101.5 (2005): 1427-1432.
5. Hagen, Kåre B., et al. "The Updated Cochrane Review of Bed Rest for Low Back Pain and Sciatica." *Spine* 30.5 (2005): 542-546.
6. Glaros, Alan G., Karen Williams, and Leonard Lausten. "The Role of Parafunctions, Emotions and Stress in Predicting Facial Pain." *The Journal of the American Dental Association* 136.4 (2005): 451-458.
7. Raymond, Isabelle, et al. "Quality of Sleep and Its Daily Relationship to Pain Intensity in Hospitalized Adult Burn Patients." *Pain* 92.3 (2001): 381-388.
8. Chou, Roger, et al. "The Effectiveness and Risks of Long-Term Opioid Therapy for Chronic Pain: a Systematic Review for a National Institutes of Health Pathways to Prevention Workshop." *Annals of Internal Medicine* 162.4 (2015): 276-286.

9. Wright, Kenneth P., et al. "Influence of Sleep Deprivation and Circadian Misalignment on Cortisol, Inflammatory Markers, and Cytokine Balance." *Brain, Behavior, and Immunity* 47 (2015): 24-34.

10. Singer, Thea. *Stress Less.* New York: Penguin Group, 2010. Print.

11. Schmitz, Gerd, and Josef Ecker. "The Opposing Effects of n-3 and n-6 Fatty Acids." *Progress in Lipid Research* 47.2 (2008): 147-155.

12. Calder, Philip C. "n- 3 Polyunsaturated Fatty Acids, Inflammation, and Inflammatory Diseases." *The American Journal of Clinical Nutrition* 83.6 (2006): S1505-1519S.

10 ADDICTION

Bill had already improved his back pain since embarking on the health journey guided by these podcasts, but he had felt even further improvement after the last episode. He truly felt in control again, and realized that his back wasn't 'broken' like he had sometimes imagined, and that he had much more influence over his pain experience than he imagined. He was paying more attention to his body, his breathing, and his hydration status. He could sense that when he slept poorly, his pain was worse the next day. He could also tell that the long hours of driving the RV were hurting his back, and that he actually craved more movement than he had realized. After speaking with Carol, they agreed to rotate driving shifts every hour, to enable each person to move around, stretch, and exercise. There was just no sense in trying to be a hero driver when it meant increased back pain for days afterwards.

Tenth Podcast

Dopamine and Addiction

Easter egg hunts. We all remember them—some of us still attend them—but perhaps we haven't thought about the relationship to dopamine and addiction before, so let's dwell on them for a moment. Imagine an egg hunt where lots of children are eagerly searching for the next egg filled with candy. They are scrambling over hills, peeking behind bushes, and are generally very motivated for that next exciting moment when they find another egg. Now imagine an Easter where there is no egg hunt. Rather, the kids wake up to find a basket next to them, simply overflowing with all sorts of candy. The children will have an immense moment of euphoria and then quickly return to baseline.

Fast forward one year, and once again the children are now engaged in an egg hunt. Only this time, the children don't seem very eager to run over that next hill, or peek behind that next bush. Each egg they find is less exciting than it was last year. It seems as if the children have lost some of their motivation and enjoyment in this once great tradition.

The Easter eggs and the candy are dopamine in this analogy, and the children could be considered addicted to candy (not a far stretch from most children, really)—the lesson being that when we engage in behaviors that flood our brains with huge amounts of dopamine like binge drinking, binge eating, drug use or sexual acts, we become less motivated to perform daily tasks like going to work, exercising, and cooking healthy meals for ourselves.[1]

This is why it is so difficult to stick to a healthy lifestyle the day after a night of drinking—our brain is craving high levels of dopamine, and foods like salads and hummus don't flood our brains with dopamine the way that foods high in fats and sugars do.

So, yet again, the lesson is moderation—how boring. Below is a list of ways to keep your dopamine levels well balanced so that you don't find yourself craving high amounts of fat and sugar, or worse, alcohol and cigarettes:

1. Make a list of the dopamine-rich activities and items in your life: gambling, caffeine, nicotine, alcohol, sweets, etc., so that you are aware of them.

2. Recognize that none of these activities are 100% off limits, but that indulging in any one of them too much will likely lead to an unbalancing of your cravings and push you off your healthy track.

3. Try to *enjoy* these dopamine-rich activities as much as possible while you're indulging in them. In other words, if you are going to eat cheesecake, do it purposefully. Chew slowly, savor the creamy consistency, relish the subtle vanilla, and truly enjoy what you are doing. The more you enjoy these delights, the less amount of them you will require to gain the satisfaction you are seeking.

4. Sprinkle your day with these activities, rather than enjoy them all in one sitting. Try having a glass of wine with lunch, rather than waiting until 9pm and then having two. The more you spread these activities throughout your day, the more balanced you will be, and you will find that your motivation is more consistent.

5. Make your weekends more like your weekdays. Common to many people is the habit of living like a saint during the week and a devil on the weekends; this is very problematic, as it completely

disrupts your dopamine balance, making you almost zombie-like come Sunday and Monday, due to the deluge of dopamine on Friday and Saturday. Try to spread these dopamine-rich activities out throughout the week, and keep your schedule as consistent as possible to optimize your focus and adherence to healthy living.

6. Don't chase the high. One of the most dangerous habits is the desire to follow up a dopamine-rich night with a dopamine-rich day. For example, waking up with a hangover, and then immediately having a 32 oz. coffee and donut. Try to let your brain slowly stabilize and regain its natural sensitivity to dopamine. By dumping yet more dopamine right back into the system it will only postpone the inevitable catatonic-like state until later, when it will be even more intense.

7. Learn to focus more on healthy, natural ways to increase dopamine, rather than substances. Enjoyable activities such as woodworking, gardening, or playing with your children will increase dopamine levels considerably, and allow you to rely less heavily on substances for these highs. Of course, any type of physical activity, including lovemaking, is welcome as well.

8. Be careful with holidays. Holidays are a wonderful time of year, filled with friends, family, drinking and celebration. But the week after these holidays can be a painful time for payback if you have over-indulged. Overeating, overdrinking, and over-celebrating can lead to the lifeless state after a holiday, making it very difficult to adhere to, let alone start on a healthy diet and lifestyle. Enjoy your friends and family and celebrate, but try to be mindful of how much food and how many drinks you consume on these days.

Nicotine and Brain Chemistry

So you want to quit smoking? Good for you. But you've heard so many stories and anecdotes of people who have succeeded and people that have failed that you are completely fed up with it. Or perhaps you're not a smoker but you know someone who is and you simply can't understand why they can't quit? Well, hopefully I can shed a bit of light on why quitting smoking is a lot more about nicotine and brain chemistry than you might have thought.

Nicotine is a highly addictive stimulant, sort of like super-caffeine. Like caffeine, high doses are lethal, but it's in that sweet spot between lethality and no effect that humans get a good buzz from it. So, naturally, nicotine makes us feel alert and buzzed, but it also suppresses our appetite. Taking cigarettes away from a person who has notoriously struggled with her weight will make it significantly harder for that person to lose weight in the short-term. Giving up something that provides one with pleasure, only to gain weight, is something that no one wants to willingly endure.

But there's more to nicotine than just stimulation and appetite suppression. Nicotine, like most drugs, releases dopamine into the brain, creating a positive feedback loop. Dopamine makes us feel good, urging us to keep inhaling. It also makes us think about the activity that gave us that dopamine, hence the actual mental obsession with having another cigarette. Dopamine helps us to focus, keeping our brain on task, similar to how we feel after drinking coffee. So after a short cigarette, our brain is lit up like a Christmas tree, and we feel good and are able to focus on whatever lies ahead.

In addition to the nicotine, smoking requires a slowing of one's breath. As mentioned in the stress chapter, slow breathing decreases anxiety. This semi-meditative activity of inhaling a cigarette, holding one's breath, and slowly exhaling, probably decreases anxiety quite effectively, especially if done several times throughout the day. Therefore, we have a focused and happy brain which also has less anxiety. We are beginning to see how amazing those little tobacco sticks really are.

The last reason that cigarettes are so difficult to quit is that because of the aforementioned effects on the brain, people begin using cigarettes as a self-prescribed reward system. After every good effort or stressful event, the smoker looks for a cigarette. They grow accustomed to living life with multiple rewards sprinkled throughout their day, and taking away something like that from anyone would cause some serious discomfort.

So in summary, cigarettes help us to lose weight, they make us feel alert, happy, less anxious, and lastly, they provide a reward system that we have control over throughout the day. While some people may be able to quit smoking "cold turkey", it makes perfect sense why so many strong-willed people struggle with this habit, when one considers the numerous effects on brain chemistry that smoking produces.

As a side note, despite the obvious short-term hurdles associated with stopping smoking, studies have shown that after only seven weeks, smokers who quit had lower levels of depression, stress, anxiety, and had improved moods over people who continued to smoke. In fact, while cigarette smoking reduces stress in the short term, smokers in general have higher levels of stress than non-smokers do.[2] So if you can make it through those first six weeks, there is light at the end of the tunnel.

A list of activities that will improve your chances of quitting smoking:[3]

1. Talk to a medical professional about pharmaceutical options. Research has shown that Varenicline (Chantix), Bupropion (Wellbutrin), and nicotine replacement therapy are all superior to placebo.[4]
2. Attend support meetings for other people who have recently quit (group behavioral therapy).
3. Work on stress-reduction activities such as slow breathing, visualizations, exercise, yoga, etc.
4. Receive individual counseling either in-person or over the phone or Internet.
5. Use the STAR method:
    a. Set a date: pick a date on the calendar for when you will quit smoking. Ideally, this will be a time when you will have minimum stress in your life and little stress on the horizon.
    b. Tell everyone: tell all of your friends and family that you are going to quit on that date, and ask them to help support you in your efforts.
    c. Assess barriers to success: Anticipate areas where quitting may be particularly hard, such as at a bar, or on a work break. By assessing these barriers to success, you can plan accordingly and be more likely to succeed.
    d. Remove all smoking paraphernalia and clean any surfaces that smell of smoke including clothing, home and car.

6. Increase your physical activity.
7. Choose healthier foods.
8. Focus on building and sustaining quality social connections with friends and family.
9. Follow the strategy for replacing unhealthy habits with healthier habits as outlined previously.

Alcohol and Its Many Barbs

I enjoy alcohol, perhaps too much from time to time. There is great joy to be gained from drinking— this I admit freely, and by no means would I ever try to discourage someone from enjoying the pleasures that this chemical has brought to humans for over 5000 years. Yet to live a balanced healthy life, it will help if we examine a few of the inherent drawbacks in this potion, lest we fall prey to them like so many others before us.

Effect on sleep: As mentioned in the chapter on sleep, alcohol ruins REM sleep. Many people can relate to the experience of drinking heavily, going to sleep, and finding ourselves awake only four hours later. Alcohol prevents us from obtaining quality REM sleep, which occurs mainly during the second half of the night. The result is a day of fogginess, poor focus and poor memory.

Effect on dopamine regulation: As mentioned above, dopamine is the critical neurotransmitter which rewards us for activities. When well balanced, we should receive natural doses of dopamine after completing tasks, making love, and eating a meal. But when we use substances like alcohol, particularly in excess, we flood our brain with dopamine. While at the time we feel good, the next day we feel like a zombie, since our brain responds to this flood by decreasing the number of dopamine receptors. Ultimately, we find it more difficult to complete everyday tasks like washing dishes and working out because our internal reward system is temporarily damaged. String together a few nights of heavy drinking and you'll find it nearly impossible to even make your bed in the morning.

Effect on appetite, blood sugar and body weight: Alcohol consumption, especially in higher doses, will trigger insulin release. This will result in a decrease in blood sugar levels and stimulate your appetite. Nothing is worse for weight gain than ingesting large amounts of food and sugar late at night. Additionally, the excess calories from drinking are not satiating the way that food is, making most people consume more calories than they need that day. The result is that overdrinking and overeating often go hand in hand. Furthermore, the long-term effect of excess drinking is actually a decrease in insulin sensitivity, which is one of the first steps towards the development of type II diabetes.

Effect on anxiety: Alcohol reduces anxiety in the short-term. This "depressant" activity of alcohol is also why it aids people in falling asleep initially. But once the alcohol is cleared from your system, the brain becomes more sensitive to anxiety than before. Turning to alcohol to calm one's nerves is a short-term solution that will only lead to long-term problems.

Effect on longevity: Obviously, long-term use of high levels of alcohol has serious negative consequences on numerous organ systems. Binge-drinking episodes probably damage the brain the most, followed by the liver, pancreas, kidneys, and nasopharyngeal tissues. In the long run, overindulgence in alcohol will tip the scales in favor of damage over repair, making your biological age look older than your chronological age.

In summary, treat alcohol with the respect it deserves. In moderation (one to three drinks per day depending on your body weight and metabolism), alcohol is your friend and can improve various health parameters. But exceed this amount by just a few drinks and be prepared for the host of unwanted negative effects that will ensue, making it all the harder to live a healthy, balanced life.

How Socialization Can Save Us

For some people, life is hard. Rather than an optimistic utopia filled with endless possibilities, life is a series of challenges with traps and obstacles littered everywhere. Over time, it can feel like life is pulling us down, and that we simply do not have the strength to resist temptations on our own. The truth is, we don't. We never will. We need support and help from family and friends because we are communal beings that gain strength from social bonds. These bonds are what keep us buoyed against the countless obstacles and challenges in life, and allow us to persist despite numerous challenges, such as addiction and failure.

These social relationships act like a support system, holding us up against the downward pull of life. By building strong social bonds, we can assume greater responsibility and become more resistant to the numerous challenges of daily life. What does this mean to people who are addicted? It means that forming strong social bonds with family and friends is the best strategy for long-term independence from addiction. Research has shown that addiction thrives in people who feel isolated and lonely. Yet place these same individuals in an environment where they feel connected to other humans, and they will have the strength to resist their addiction and break free from their chemical dependency.[5] In other words, people often turn to drugs and other chemicals when they lack quality social connections. When these social connections are reformed, however, the individual no longer has the same desire to use drugs and chemicals, because the relationships they now have provide that feeling of connection and happiness that the drugs used to provide.

The bottom line is that our environment, specifically the quality of our social connections, serves as both a protective barrier to addiction, and the most proven method of escape for current addicts. Therefore, focusing less on which chemical should be used to wean someone off a street drug, and more on building quality relationships, will be the best strategy towards overcoming addiction and becoming a healthy and independent person for the future.

Bill and Carol's Thoughts

Bill paid close attention to this most recent podcast. While he had fortunately not developed any overt addictions in his life, he certainly understood the desire to seek dopamine-rich activities in his life. Particularly difficult for him was resisting the temptation on Friday to overindulge in pizza and beer. After working hard for five days, Bill had always looked forward to pizza night, where he could drink multiple beers, have dessert, and sleep in late on Saturday. But waking up on Saturday required a huge coffee and usually some sweets to get him going again, and he was never as productive as he wanted to be. Then, when Monday came along, getting out of bed was a chore. Now that he was retired, there was no reason for his weekends to differ dramatically from his weekdays, and sprinkling those dopamine-rich activities throughout the week should not prove too difficult for him, and should help him stay focused on being healthy.

Carol, on the other hand, had long struggled with holidays. She had undertaken numerous diets over the years, yet when the holidays came she had usually fallen apart. Now, after listening to this podcast, she realized just how devastating the overindulging was to her willpower and her brain chemistry. Once you had a huge meal with alcohol and sugar and sweets, it could form a feedback cycle, leaving you craving more the next day. Being tempted by cookies and cakes for multiple days, while drinking champagne, wine, and other spirits, had set the stage for a month of sin and indulgence that could undo all of the healthy habits she had worked so hard to form. Carol knew that this holiday season she would have a plan, and would make sure to break up those days of indulgence with days of moderation. Also, she would try to indulge earlier in the day, and avoid excess carbs and alcohol in the evening.

Despite neither Carol nor Bill having any problem with cigarettes or nicotine products over the years, they certainly had friends who had struggled to kick the habit. After hearing all of the hurdles inherent in overcoming this addiction, they felt more compassion for their friends. They realized that support was far more important than preaching and chastising, and that sharing this podcast might kickstart them onto the path of freedom from nicotine. Even more interesting was learning how nicotine affects the brain, serving almost like a medication to certain people, allowing them to function at a high level in their jobs and in social settings.

As the weeks on their health journey continued for Bill and Carol, they realized how interconnected all of their actions were. Each facet of their health, be it willpower, or sleep, or anxiety, was intricately connected to other facets, relying on a unified approach to improving one's health. It appeared that the same was true of addiction, that in order to overcome it, one needed to address multiple facets of one's health in order to improve all of the interconnected pieces that contributed to and maintained the unhealthy addiction.

References

1. Bello, Nicholas T., and Andras Hajnal. "Dopamine and Binge Eating Behaviors." *Pharmacology Biochemistry and Behavior* 97.1 (2010): 25-33.
2. Parrott, Andy C. "Does Cigarette Smoking Cause Stress?" *American Psychologist* 54.10 (1999): 817.
3. Lemmens, Valery, et al. "Effectiveness of Smoking Cessation Interventions among Adults: a Systematic Review of Reviews." *European Journal of Cancer Prevention* 17.6 (2008): 535-544.
4. Wu, Ping, et al. "Effectiveness of Smoking Cessation Therapies: a Systematic Review and Meta-Analysis." *BMC Public Health* 6.1 (2006): 300.
5. Hari, Johann. *Chasing the Scream: The First and Last Days of the War on Drugs.* Bloomsbury Publishing USA, 2015.

11 HAPPINESS

By now, Bill and Carol were truly seeing the rewards of their dedication and commitment to the health principles detailed in the podcasts. Without having to sacrifice any specific food or spend money on overly-processed specialty items, they had lost over ten pounds in the last ten weeks and felt better than they had in years. Bill's back pain was infrequent and short-lived. Carol was cooking more and spending more time outdoors on gardening and farming than ever before. They had more energy and less stress, which led to more time enjoying each other and their children, and less time taking naps and worrying about things beyond their control. They had both avoided cholesterol-lowering drugs, as their muscle mass increased and their fat mass decreased. They looked healthier, were more active, and were content and happy. They viewed the future with optimism.

Eleventh Podcast

Pleasure Versus Well-Being

I think it's safe to assume that all humans want to be happy. If that is true, then why do numerous people try to achieve happiness through such diverse means? In addition to those trying to achieve happiness, it seems that even more people are utterly confused about where to even begin to find happiness.

Much of this confusion centers around what happiness means. Let's discuss the differences between the momentary pleasures of life and the longer-lasting concept of well-being.

We are all familiar with pleasures. These are the id-based urges such as hunger, thirst, sexual desire, etc. They operate primarily through the dopamine system, giving us a feeling of temporary satisfaction and happiness. Whether it be snorting cocaine, eating chocolate, playing a video game, binge-drinking, or having sex, they all flood our system with dopamine and provide us with the very desirable feeling of pleasure. But is this what we mean when we speak of happiness?

I think we should contrast these momentary pleasures, many of which are addictive, with the less intense but longer-lasting concept of well-being. If kindling are the pleasures, then the larger log that really keeps the fire burning is the well-being in one's life.

Well-being is the overall emotional state that we find ourselves in day to day. Well-being is the experience of minimal anxiety, low tension, overall good health, and a feeling of general satisfaction. Well-being is something that washes over us slowly, and lingers, making us feel like everything is going to be alright. One could imagine that a monk or other ascetic person might feel this calm easiness in his life often. While well-being doesn't require a complete removal of momentary pleasures, a person with high well-being doesn't seek them out as an end in themselves. Rather, a person with well-being most likely feels part of something larger than himself, and has a greater purpose to his life than mere physical pleasures.

If happiness is just a series of physical pleasures strung together, than hooking our brain up to the matrix and allowing a computer program to stimulate dopamine release could be the solution to a happy life. But few people would agree that this is the true nature of happiness. I argue that well-being is very close to what most people agree that happiness is, and the process of obtaining it is far more complicated than merely flooding our brain with dopamine temporarily.

Temporary Happiness Versus Long-Term Satisfaction

Continuing the theme of short versus long-term happiness, we now turn our attention to satisfaction.

As humans, most of us crave challenges. We love challenges because we have learned that the harder the struggle, the sweeter the victory. Some of us become nearly obsessed with the pursuit of challenges, engaging in risky or dangerous behavior such as climbing Mount Everest or kayaking across an ocean. Despite weeks or even months of discomfort during the process, we are rewarded with an overwhelmingly sweet happiness upon accomplishment of the goal. The winning Super Bowl team is very happy indeed, but how long does this last?

You see, if we put happiness at the top of the pyramid as the ultimate goal, then why would we spend months of discomfort only to receive a few days' or a few weeks' worth of happiness? Is the habit of setting goals and achieving them sufficient to satisfy the desire for a satisfied life?

When psychologists discuss happiness they often break it into two distinct phases: momentary happiness, and long-term satisfaction with one's life. While I feel that both are important, it is necessary to distinguish between the two. While accomplishing a goal or seeking physical pleasure will both result in a high momentary happiness, these are short-lived by definition. And there are countless goals in the world that either cannot be achieved or will result in failure far short of the finish line, leaving us with an absence of happiness if that is the only purpose. But by focusing less on momentary happiness and more on long-term satisfaction, we may be able to create a better sense of well-being that doesn't rely so heavily on goals and dopamine levels.

Long-term satisfaction is difficult to achieve, but let's look at the infamous Steve Jobs as an example of how we may better achieve it. If we assume that his biographies are fairly accurate, then we can safely characterize Steve as a relentless narcissist and perfectionist, whose quest for producing excellent products overshadowed his attention to his family and health. While he was clearly a genius with unparalleled achievements, it was only later in life when Steve admitted regret over the way he'd treated his friends and family. I can't comment on Steve's short or long-term happiness, but I will use his life as an example of someone who reveled in achieving goals, rather than promoting those parts of his life that might lead to long-term satisfaction.

I will end this discussion with the eulogy versus résumé comparison that several authors before me have raised. We can choose to create an amazing résumé, replete with the most remarkable accomplishments like Steve Jobs, or we can choose to create a life that will be remembered by a beautiful eulogy, and have family and friends who will talk fondly of us for years to come. I am not telling you which path is correct, but I am fairly confident which way will lead to long-term satisfaction and which one towards temporary happiness.

Higher Orders of Happiness

There are roughly four orders, or levels, of happiness. The first order is something we've previously touched upon: dopamine surges. This level includes the vast majority of daily experiences and pleasures that humans seek, including eating, sex, cocaine, roller-coasters, receiving an A on a test, winning a chess game, buying a new car, etc. While fairly intense at the time, they fade quickly and rarely make us feel larger than ourselves. This order of happiness relies on the same basic pleasures that are available to most animals, and while it feels good at the time, it pales in comparison to the higher levels.

Love, or more accurately, being in love—this is second order happiness. While still relying on dopamine initially, there are more chemicals involved, such as oxytocin, which create richer and more complicated feelings of happiness. This level includes not only romantic love, but also platonic love and maternal love. The feeling a mother has when breastfeeding her child is an elevated happiness that rises above mere dopamine-pleasures. Likewise, being in love gives life a glow, making every day seem like a gift. Love is a very special form of happiness, but there are orders even higher than love.

Sacrifice, philanthropy, and charity on a grand scale—as good as love feels, the feeling one receives when sacrificing oneself, or giving of oneself to a larger purpose or great number of people, is even higher than love. I am describing someone who donates his kidney to a stranger, or a grandfather selling his favorite car so that his granddaughter may attend college. Larger still, I am referring to hunger strikers like Gandhi, who are sacrificing for a larger purpose. While physically they may be in tremendous discomfort or pain, they have transcended the happiness that is confined to their physical body or to a two-person relationship, and have entered the realm where their actions may now contribute to numerous people's happiness in a deeply profound way. While this may appear to be the pinnacle of human happiness, there lies one more realm with an even loftier experience.

Spiritual enlightenment. It doesn't matter whether you're religious or atheistic, this can take on many forms. From the monk who achieves this while meditating, to the astrophysicist who experiences it while pondering the multiverse, it is an experience which takes place outside of ourselves. It is something that transcends our physical bodies, and even our human race, to encompass the entire universe. For a moment, we tap into a deep-seated knowledge and subconscious instinct that long lie dormant. We momentarily feel at one with the universe, with all that is in existence around us, and concepts such as the individual fade from importance. This enlightenment is the hardest to achieve and is rarely achieved by average people. It takes dedication, and focus, and a keen sense of balance to touch this rarified realm. Yet it is the most glorious emotional state that human beings are capable of achieving to date... one that should give us perspective when we think the world is just a search for our next dopamine rush.

Depression and Control

I know a thing or two about depression, having had several bouts of it throughout my life. After experimenting with a few different pharmaceuticals, I decided to use my own personal strategies to deal with my mental ups and downs. But regardless of which method each individual chooses to manage his or her own personal struggles, the theme that underlies most episodes of depression is *control*.

Depression is really the result of feeling helpless, of feeling that your actions no longer have any impact on the world around you. Depression can be induced in rats by shocking them without any means of stopping the shock. Within a short period of time the rats become depressed so that when you do provide a lever which, when pressed, would cease the shock, they no longer attempt to press it.[1] Instead, the rats merely sit in the corner, accepting the shocks, and accepting their fate. They have learned that their actions no longer matter, and so they have given up.

Similarly, humans are equally susceptible to this condition when placed in an environment where we have no control. Whether it be a job where our actions don't matter, or an abusive relationship where our partner ignores all of our efforts to resist, we can quickly find ourselves like the rat in the cage, depressed and defeated.

The solution, while not easy, is to focus only on those things in your life over which you have complete control. For example, when feeling depressed, simply make a list of everything in your life over which you have complete control. This may sound silly at first, but if done in earnest, I assure you that the feeling of helplessness will subside some, simply by making this list. It is important while composing this list to not skip any items, no matter how small they may seem. This may include items like: when I choose to brush my teeth, when I choose to go to bed, what music I choose to listen to on my commute to work, etc. The more items you list, the less helpless you will feel, as you begin to notice just how many things you have control over in your life. While adjusting your bedtime or commute music may not change your life overnight, focusing on those areas in your life that you actually have real control over will make you feel empowered once again.

Ultimately, removing yourself from oppressive and abusive situations is also imperative; I am not implying that making a list can somehow make domestic violence tolerable. Yet, we often know that we need to remove ourselves from bad situations but feel helpless to do anything initially. It is by making this list, and focusing on our controllable areas, that we begin to counter the inertia and gain the momentum that is required to make difficult changes. I am a strong believer in the power of counselors and pharmaceuticals in the battle against depression, but in the meantime, empower yourself for free by focusing on the things that you *do* control in your life, rather than becoming frustrated over the things you *do not.*

Happiness, Health, and Relationships

We can all agree that most people would like happiness, health, and good relationships in their life. Millions of songs are written about love, billions of dollars are spent on health-related products, and millions of hours are spent talking to counselors and taking drugs to restore happiness to us. Yet, these three goals all have one thing in common that seems to elude even the smartest of people: hard work.

I think the connection between hard work and good relationships is fairly familiar to us. Married couples celebrating their 50th anniversary are often asked what the "secret" is to their relationship and the answer is often "hard work." Yet despite knowing that, countless people continue to search for the magic bullet to a great relationship. We often spend lots of money and time on eHarmony and other websites, using complicated algorithms to find the "perfect match" for us. Regardless of how perfect your partner is, hard work will still be required. I know finding a partner who stays beautiful forever, never criticizes us, never expects us to change, and is always sexually hungry sounds like a surefire plan, but the truth is far more sobering.

Despite good health requiring hard work as well, it seems that people simply cannot resist the allure of finding some magic pill or easy solution that will give them perfect health on a platter, without the hassle of having to work hard for it. People search for the "perfect food," the "perfect exercise," the "perfect diet," as if once these are found they can merely hit cruise control and enjoy great health indefinitely. As outlined in this book, great health is the result of a series of behaviors which, over time, lead to a healthier you. There is no fast-track or easy button to press and then relax. We must put effort in every day, and eventually we will be rewarded.

Happiness is the same deal. We are all looking for a one-time decision or behavior that will create happiness. Some people think that if we abandon our civilized life and live like monks then we'll be happy. Or if we become doctors and make $250K a year, then we'll be happy. Or, if we find the perfect partner and get married, then we'll be happy. But none of these will result in long-term happiness. There is no one single event or behavior that will bring us a happiness that will last. Happiness, like health and good relationships, requires hard work every day to achieve and maintain. Over time, it will become easier to perform the actions that will bring us good health, great relationships, and long-lasting happiness.

But this is good news, because it means that it is never too late to start righting the ship. Since these long-sought ideals are found on a daily basis, we can start acting differently today, and can find that all three of these may come to us overnight. Anything valuable should be worth the effort, and what is more valuable than loving relationships, good health, and happiness? If you aren't willing to work hard for these goals, then they'll remain just distant dreams, not based on reality. But on the other hand, if you are willing to work hard every day, then you will obtain what you want and live a truly wonderful life in the process. Good luck!

A list of activities that have been shown to improve happiness:[2]

1. Give money and time to help those less fortunate than you.[3]
2. Be present in the moment, rather than daydreaming about elsewhere or keeping your phone on the table during a meal.[4]
3. Take time each day to think about three things for which you are truly grateful.
4. Perform a job or hobby where you are able to get into "the zone" on a regular basis. In other words, a mindset where you aren't even thinking, but are sort of acting on instinct and nearly everything you do is correct and effective. Think of Michael Jordan during the NBA finals as an example.[5]
5. Be around people with whom you have a connection or bond.
6. Be around people with similar interests and values.
7. Be part of something larger than yourself.
8. Only concern yourself with areas of your life over which you have control.

Bill and Carol's Thoughts

The past 11 weeks were at first unfamiliar and

scary, but now the journey was almost over. The whole time it never felt like hard work, or sacrifice, but rather a realigning of their lives with the way they knew they should have been living from the beginning. Now, it seemed like everything they were working hard for was finally coming together. The whole goal of life is to be happy, satisfied, and content. Health is really just a piece of life, one that when it is good makes you more likely to be happy. But health is not the end in itself, but rather a means to the end, which is loving life and living every moment to the fullest.

The sections on temporary versus long-term and pleasure versus well-being were really reinforcements to the way Bill and Carol had been living their life anyway. Throughout the past three months, they had learned to use willpower to resist indulging in high-dopamine activities and to enjoy the longer lasting moments that improved their well-being. Likewise, they had focused their attention on the present moment by slowing their breathing and performing more activities with purpose, such as gardening and farming, rather than focusing on far-away goals that required long bouts of detachment from the present moment.

The eulogy analogy was particularly helpful for Carol in explaining how she thought about her life. She agreed wholeheartedly that building quality relationships with friends and family was more important than how much money you had in your bank account when you died. She had started this health journey as a means to ensure that she would be alive to see her grandchildren graduate from college. Now she was realizing that this journey was about much more than just health, but rather about the way she lived her life. She realized that health and happiness are intricately connected, and trying to become healthier while being depressed would be ineffective. Health is a result of how you live your life, not a formula or diet that you follow. A happy, active person, low in stress, well-rested, and at peace with herself is likely to be a healthy person as well. It made sense now why every diet and weight loss book prior to this had been unsuccessful: they had failed to address the "other" components in a person's life, and had just focused either on diet, or exercise, without addressing happiness, sleep, or stress levels.

Bill enjoyed the section on depression and control. Their youngest son had battled with depression for years, finally finding some stability after he'd married. Yet Bill had often found it difficult to empathize with his son and didn't know exactly what to say or how to help him. After hearing depression so simply explained, he felt more capable of relating to his son should he encounter another bout of depression in the future. At least now Bill could refer him to this podcast in the hopes that something he heard could be useful to him the way it had been to Bill. Bill even thought back to his parenting style with his son and wondered if giving his son a bit more control over decisions as a child would have made a difference in his level of depression as an adult. While not one to dwell on the past, it did make him think differently about his grandchildren and he would keep an eye out for the early signs of depression should it afflict them as well.

Carol and Bill had both felt intimidated by the part about spiritual enlightenment. While they had both recently started attending church again, and had undertaken slow breathing on a daily basis, they admitted that they never thought about achieving enlightenment in any real way. They thought that a more realistic goal might be to start volunteering their time and sacrificing a bit of their money to help people less fortunate than themselves. They figured that if they could first achieve the third level of happiness, then they could start to worry about achieving the highest level. They both agreed that they had enough free time in retirement to donate a few hours each week to helping those less fortunate, and they knew that their church would have many opportunities lined up for them to become engaged quickly. While it didn't initially seem as rewarding as falling in love, they trusted the process and believed that their volunteering could quickly become a very meaningful piece of their life.

References

1. Weiss, Jay M., et al. "Behavioral Depression Produced by an Uncontrollable Stressor: Relationship to Norepinephrine, Dopamine, and Serotonin Levels in Various Regions of Rat Brain." *Brain Research Reviews* 3.2 (1981): 167-205.
2. Layous, Kristin, and Sonja Lyubomirsky. "The How, Why, What, When, and Who of Happiness: Mechanisms Underlying the Success of Positive Activity Interventions." *Positive Emotion: Integrating the Light Sides and Dark Sides* (2014): 473-495.
3. Sääksjärvi, Maria, et al. "In the Long Run, Other-Focused Happiness-Boosting Activities Are More Effective than Self-Focused Activities." *E-European Advances in Consumer Research Volume 10* (2013).
4. Baer, Ruth A. *Practising Happiness: How Mindfulness Can Free You from Psychological Traps and Help You Build the Life You Want.* Hachette UK, 2014.
6. Csikszentmihalyi, Mihaly. *Flow: The Psychology of Happiness.* Random House, 2013.

12 A TYPICAL DAY IN THE LIFE OF BILL AND CAROL

Bill and Carol wake up at 6:30 to the sound of an old-school alarm clock they placed across the room. Carol prefers this, since it allows her to completely turn her phone off each night—plus, she has to get up to turn it off, and this prevents her from undergoing the needless activity of snoozing. They wake early, as they find it allows them to accomplish more tasks throughout the day, and makes them feel more productive.

Bill starts grinding the coffee, and proceeds to pour the hot water into his French press to start the morning. Carol waters her plants and takes her dog for a walk. She has decided to use this time to practice her slow breathing each day.

Bill and Carol sit down to enjoy their coffee and enjoy a pastry that Carol baked yesterday. This is the time for them to enjoy their sweets, and they do so wholeheartedly. They also listen to a podcast together. Since they have finished the health journey podcast, they now listen to a new podcast focusing more on the research behind behavioral change. It discusses the newest evidence in the field of health behavior and health psychology and how to most effectively change one's habits. They had grown fond of their weekly podcasts and now have a different podcast to listen to each morning. It is more relaxing and less expensive than reading the paper, and they can move around and clean dishes while listening so they don't have to be stuck at the table the whole time.

Carol cleans the dishes while Bill does a few maintenance exercises for his back. Then Carol decides to pick some vegetables from the garden for tonight's dinner. Bill uses this time to get ready in the bathroom and do his slow breathing exercises while shaving, brushing his teeth, etc.

After his breathing exercises, Bill decides to work on the wooden chairs that he is going to give to his son as a birthday present. Bill has really enjoyed his quiet time in the garage working with his hands and on a gift to his children. He remembers to bring his water bottle with him, filled with a lightly carbonated low calorie drink so that he can stay hydrated.

Carol finishes up in the garden and decides to call her sister and make sure that her visit to the farm next week is still on schedule. Carol has been spending more time with her sister and more time on the farm since listening to the podcast. She also keeps her water bottle nearby with her, drinking more than she feels she needs to maintain adequate hydration, especially since it's cool outside.

After Carol and Bill finish up with their activities, they prepare for lunch. They are having leftover pizza that they made yesterday. It was whole grain dough they picked up with fresh mozzarella, tomatoes and basil and garlic from their garden, and some uncured pork belly from Carol's sister's farm. They accompany this with a small salad of arugula and carrots and balsamic vinaigrette. Bill and Carol love wine, and they enjoy a bottle of a refreshing white wine from Northern Italy with their meal.

After lunch Bill likes to take a 20 minute nap, and Carol is there to make sure he didn't oversleep. As long as he awakes after 20 minutes, he feels refreshed, rather than groggy.

Carol goes in the kitchen again, putting together a fresh coleslaw of carrots and cabbage from her garden. She is bringing this to the church potluck they hold every Thursday. Carol and Bill attend mass at 5pm, followed by the potluck, at which they make sure to only eat until they feel full. They are there more for the social aspect, and less for the food, as their lunch was the biggest meal of the day anyway. They try to keep the amount of carbs at this point in the evening to a minimum, and instead focus on the proteins and vegetables. They still sample nearly everything, but keep the portions of sweets on the small side. Again, they each enjoy a glass of wine with their meal, knowing they have more than two hours before bedtime for their bodies to process it.

After the potluck, Carol provides tutoring services to children at the local school, and Bill referees the basketball league. They have enjoyed being busy throughout the day and feel connected to their community through these activities.

Later in the evening they walk the dog together, talk about the day, and review the things for which they are grateful.

Before going to bed, Bill and Carol consult their checklists. First on the list is hydration, so they make sure they have drunk enough water to avoid waking up with a desert mouth in the middle of the night. Next, they both use the bathroom to ensure they won't wake up to relieve themselves in the middle of the night. Next, they silence their phones and set their old-fashioned alarm. Carol has a mild skin cream she applies to certain parts of her skin to help keep her skin problems at bay. Bill has a CPAP machine that he wears to prevent sleep apnea. Bill also uses a sleep mask to help him to fall asleep, while Carol needs some ambient noise to help her fall asleep. After completing their respective checklists, they are prepared for a luxurious night's rest, which is the best way to prepare for their next amazing day!

ADDITIONAL READINGS

Diet

- Pollan, Michael. *In Defense of Food: An Eater's Manifesto.* Penguin, 2008.
- Davis, William. *Wheat Belly: Lose the Wheat, Lose the Weight, and Find Your Path Back to Health.* Rodale, 2014.

Habits

- Duhigg, Charles. *The Power of Habit: Why We Do What We Do in Life and Business.* Vol. 34. No. 10. Random House, 2012.

Addiction

- Wilson, Bill. *Alcoholics Anonymous: Big Book.* AA World Services, 2015.

Willpower

- McGonigal, Kelly. *The Willpower Instinct: How Self-Control Works, Why it Matters, and What You Can Do to Get More of It.* Penguin, 2011.

Stress

- Brown, Richard P., and P. Gerbarg. *The Healing Power of the Breath.* Boston, MA: Shambhala, 2012.

Sleep

- Stevenson, Shawn. *Sleep Smarter: 21 Proven Tips to Sleep Your Way To a Better Body, Better Health and Bigger Success.* San Bernardino, CA: Self Published, 2014.

Weight loss industry

- Schwartz, Robert M. *Diets Don't Work 3rd edition.* Houston, TX: Breakthru Publishing, 1996.

Disease

- Buettner, Dan. *The Blue Zones Solution: Lessons for Living Longer from the People Who've Lived the Longest.* Washington, D.C.: National Geographic Society, 2015.
- Friedman, Howard, and Leslie R. Martin. *The Longevity Project: Surprising Discoveries for Health and Long Life from the Landmark Eight Decade Study.* Hay House, Inc, 2011.
- Sarno, John E. *Healing Back Pain: The Mind-Body Connection.* Grand Central Publishing, 2001.

Happiness

- Gilbert, Daniel. *Stumbling on Happiness.* Vintage Canada, 2009.

ABOUT THE AUTHOR

Jesse is a lifelong student of health. A graduate of the University of New Hampshire and the University of Connecticut, he has accumulated over 11 years of undergraduate and graduate level coursework. He is a licensed physical therapist, a former medical student, an author of numerous academic papers on a variety of health-related topics, a former Certified Strength and Conditioning Specialist, and a prolific lecturer.

Jesse's diverse education, including both clinical and laboratory experiences, allows him to detect patterns and connections between disparate health topics. His ability to use analogies to explain complicated health principles enables quicker understanding by his students, leading to rapid adoption of his principles.

Jesse is the CEO and founder of LangLife, a health and wellness company. He currently resides in Torrington, CT, with his family.